Excellence in Compassionate Nursing Care
LEADING THE CHANGE

CLAIRE CHAMBERS

*Leader, Specialist Community Public Health Nursing
and Community Specialist Practice Programmes
Oxford Brookes University*

and

ELAINE RYDER

*Formerly, Leader, Community Specialist
Practice Nursing Programmes
Oxford Brookes University
Now working for Age UK*

Foreword by
SARAH H KAGAN PhD, RN
*Lucy Walker Honorary Term Professor of
Gerontological Nursing, School of Nursing
Clinical Nurse Specialist, Abramson Cancer Center
University of Pennsylvania, Philadelphia, PA, USA*

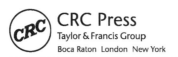

CRC Press
Taylor & Francis Group
Boca Raton London New York

CRC Press is an imprint of the
Taylor & Francis Group, an **informa** business

Radcliffe Publishing Ltd
33–41 Dallington Street
London
EC1V 0BB
United Kingdom

www.radcliffepublishing.com

British Library Cataloguing in Publication Data

A catalogue record for this book is available from the British Library.

ISBN-13: 978 184619 399 6

The paper used for the text pages of this book
is FSC® certified. FSC (The Forest Stewardship
Council®) is an international network to promote
responsible management of the world's forests.

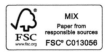

Typeset by Darkriver Design, Auckland, New Zealand

Contents

Foreword

'I'll tell you what you need to do! You need to stop talking about not using restraints and come work a night shift with me and get hit and kicked by my patients!' Her voice raged, and venomous anger arced from the nurse's eyes from the back of the cold auditorium right to the front, where I stood trying to complete a workshop on care for acutely ill older people. I was half a world away from home, facing a nurse exuding the anger and helplessness I observe so often wherever I go in the world. There I stood, my pulse racing and my face flushing, frozen for a moment. I barely contained my own emotions – perhaps I did not even achieve that and tell myself I did to soften the pain of this interaction – and knew I had only a moment in which to respond lest I lose the entire group of sixty or so nurses to the despair of helplessness and anger about their practice.

My own emotions churned with shock, frustration, pain, sadness and pity. Shock – that this nursing colleague responded with only anger and disdain to discussion of evidence-based techniques to manage delirium and agitation that I have personally experienced as effective. Frustration – that I could not reach this colleague with reasoned evidence to improve patient care. Pain – that I was unable to convey my own practice in a manner that resonated with her perspective, allowing her to hear the knowledge I shared. I had indeed faced very similar nights filled with agitated, discomforted and distressed patients; those nights live in my memory and my dreams, driving me to find a better way to care for such patients. Sadness – that this colleague conveyed an image of patients – ill, frail older people mired in delirium – as the enemy. How, I wondered, has nursing practice come to this place? Pity – that this or any colleague would and could feel so lacking in power and ability to care for any patient, any person in need of nursing care. Shock, frustration, pain, sadness and pity are emotions I expect nurses to assuage in their patients and family members. Observing such powerfully helpless and negative emotions among my nursing colleagues is for me a sharp sign that our profession is perhaps veering offtrack.

Veering offtrack suggests to me that we are losing focus on fundamental aspects of care and on the provision of that care with compassion. Patients and their families tell us in so many ways that they value and indeed require compassionate care. Nursing care is, in many ways, no longer rote care without compassion. In the worst case, care without compassion is a series of actions done to a vulnerable person, stripping away personhood, dignity, humanity. The patient certainly bears this non-care. The nurse too I think suffers, as do the nurse's colleagues and co-workers. The non-care that results when compassion is absent catalyzes a vacuum of personhood, dignity and humanity that is devoid of moral direction and ethical actions. Care delivered without compassion risks the singular interaction with a particular patient while permeating others in proximity and adjacent encounters. Non-care ripples out from that original interaction, invading the thoughts and actions of other nurses, members of the care team, patients and families. Much is at risk when compassion is lost. Some form of leadership is required that we regain our balance.

How then are we specifically to regain equipoise and return to fundamentals of care and provision of compassionate care? Neither I nor Claire Chambers and Elaine Ryder are among the first to note that compassionate care is successful care, demanded by society and valued by nurses and colleagues in other disciplines alike. To be sure, none in nursing intended to lose compassion and deliver that non-care that is done to and not with or for people in need. None of our colleagues in medicine, social work, physiotherapy or other professions believes that care is possible if nurses lose compassion. As Claire Chambers and Elaine Ryder note, in this, their second book on compassionate care, if nurses do not lead to restore compassion in care, then who will do so? In fact, we must lead.

The pressing questions of regaining our balance and restoring compassion are, I find, the subject of many conversations and manuscripts. Here in America, we are all talking about patient- and family-centered care. I admit we are a bit behind in this conversation, as person-centered care has long been discussed in the United Kingdom and elsewhere. In many places, nursing is also talking about leadership – leadership for patient- or person-centered care, for excellence in care, for coordination and transitions. An important shortcoming befalls most of what I hear and read about care and leadership. It all lacks specificity and direction. We talk about centering care around the person and speak to nursing leadership for excellence, but rarely do we explicate what is necessary to achieve of what we speak. Excellence, care and leadership exist as formless concepts, too large to use in the daily rigors of nursing practice.

The nurse who challenged me in the lecture hall embodies what all of us feel at some moment and many nurses live every day. Her rage at me, at her dependent patients, and at her health-care system illustrates the likely growing sense among nurses that they are controlled by others and not in control of situations in which they can exert the power of compassion and knowledge to help others. The nurse who surprised me with her outrage exemplified the disillusionment, disempowerment and deep anger that Claire Chambers and Elaine Ryder observe is too common in our time. Many nurses experience this poignant triad when, time after time, the context for care feels barren of the time, support and structure necessary to care. I admit in hindsight that her emotion overwhelmed me and my leadership was less than I wished. I believe her outburst was a somewhat prickly request for help as much as it was a rebuke. I regret to this day that I found no better response than challenging her to imagine that an outcome other than a battle with patients was possible. I urged her to try my approach while reconsidering her despair of nursing, patients and hospitals. I missed the chance to provide some of what Claire Chambers and Elaine Ryder offer in abundance: the chance to provide forthright leadership and clear direction to regain compassion and re-establish compassionate care.

In *Excellence in Compassionate Nursing Care: leading the change*, Claire Chambers and Elaine Ryder achieve a rare synthesis of diverse works in nursing, management and leadership and an apropos distillation of elements that ground leadership to achieve excellence in compassionate care. Their treatise is direct and practical as much as it is inspiring and reassuring. In this manual for nursing leadership in our time, Claire and Elaine offer the guidance that all nurses need sometimes and some of us need now in an effort to restore that which is undoubtedly requisite for all care – the ultimately human sensibility of compassion.

Sarah H Kagan PhD, RN
Lucy Walker Honorary Term Professor of
Gerontological Nursing, School of Nursing
Clinical Nurse Specialist, Abramson Cancer Center
University of Pennsylvania, Philadelphia, PA, USA
January 2012

Preface

We are passionately interested in the importance of nursing values and believe that excellence in compassionate nursing care lies at the heart of nursing practice. We have found from writing our first book, *Compassion and Caring in Nursing,*[*] that nurses are concerned and do want to discuss and address issues when patients or clients feel that they are not being cared for with compassion.

We have spoken at numerous conferences and discussed key issues with practitioners who want to make changes in their practice areas. Sometimes they feel in a position to make these changes, and sometimes they do not, depending perhaps on how they see themselves within the hierarchy of their organisation, or whether they know how to maximise their influence within their organisation or practice area. Many nurses feel disillusioned, powerless and angry and feel that they are not valued in their roles. Often they are criticised by patients, carers, managers and colleagues as they try to carry out care in severely under-resourced circumstances.

We feel strongly that in any nursing team, every person has a role in influencing good practice, in challenging practice that is not ideal and in taking practice forward. You do not have to have 'manager' in your job title to do this – everyone has a role in leadership, and the best ideas often come from those who are in direct day-to-day contact with patients.

This book is about how to take that lead in practice, even when staffing levels are low and there are other resource constraints.

In our first book, we identified key elements in the therapeutic compassionate relationship and also the challenges that nurses face in delivering compassionate care. The challenges include resource limitations in these financially constrained times; we believe these can be addressed through clear strategies and strong leadership. Individual nurse attitude and the culture of

---

* Chambers C, Ryder E. *Compassion and Caring in Nursing.* Oxford: Radcliffe Publishing; 2009.

the practice environment are the other two challenges; again, these can be addressed by practitioners who genuinely put compassionate care at the centre of their professional role. Nurses can become role models and leaders in their organisation by increasing the level of compassionate care where they work, and their influence can spread out to nearby practice areas, like ripples from a stone thrown into a pond.

Having the confidence to be an agent for change can be a challenge, and we decided to write a book to help those who want to make that vital difference in relation to compassionate care. The chapters in this book focus on the potential challenges to compassionate care and on ways of taking a leadership role in making a positive difference, whatever your position within your nursing organisation.

There is no doubt that patients and clients, and their families and friends, value nurses who are caring and compassionate, and that is why our first book focused on case studies from the patient's or client's perspective.

We planned this book along similar lines by using case studies to make the discussion as accessible and user friendly as possible. The focus is on the integration of theory and practice throughout. We want readers to be challenged by the points for reflection, in terms of their own practice, and to recognise the dilemmas raised in the case studies. We hope that this style of writing will encourage practitioners to review their current practice and take a lead in bringing about change within their practice environment.

For us, excellence in compassionate nursing care is the key to nursing practice, and leadership is key to making this happen. Each chapter focuses on one of the challenges to compassionate care and how nurses can take a lead to address this challenge. Theory and practice are integrated by means of a case scenario that is revisited throughout the chapter. We have included numerous points for practice to generate discussion and challenge practitioners in their leadership of nursing care.

We hope that all practitioners will feel sufficiently valued and empowered to make that vital difference in relation to a patient's or client's experience of care.

Claire Chambers
Elaine Ryder
January 2012

About the authors

Claire Chambers MSc, PgDip (Prof) Ed, CPT, HV (Dip), RGN

Claire worked as a nurse in various hospital environments and then moved into health visiting. She was a health visitor, community practice teacher and lecturer–practitioner before she moved into full-time education. During her teaching career, she worked with preregistration, post-qualification and post-graduate students from various community and acute settings, but her prime interests have always been in relation to community practice. Patient- and client-centred care, diversity and cultural competence, public health and caring for people with long-term conditions, are her special interests. With Elaine Ryder, she co-authored *Compassion and Caring in Nursing*, which reflects her belief in the centrality of compassion and excellent communication skills in nursing. She has ensured that advanced communication skills and values, based care, focusing on positive attitudes to patients and clients, are central tenets of the Specialist Community Public Health Nursing and Community Specialist Practice programmes at Oxford Brookes University.

Elaine Ryder MSc, BA, DNT, RNT, Cert Ed, CPT, DN, RGN

During her nursing career, Elaine has worked in different parts of the UK as a district nurse, community practice teacher and manager and educator within primary care. Throughout this time, her particular experience and interest has been in meeting the needs of vulnerable people and their carers at home – for example, older people, people with long-term conditions, and those with palliative care or end-of-life needs – as well as caring for those with acute healthcare needs at home. She now works as an associate lecturer at Oxford Brookes University and as a flexible carer for Age UK for older people with mental health needs. Sensitive person-centred compassionate practice has always been for her the essence of nursing. The opportunity to co-author their first book, *Compassion and Caring in Nursing*, with her colleague Claire, has given her the chance to examine the truly positive impact compassionate care has on patients and clients and the opportunity to share this with others.

Acknowledgements

We would like to thank all those who have shown an interest in compassion as the central tenet of nursing.

Our patients, clients and students have always motivated us, and discussion with other healthcare professionals has also stimulated debate on this key aspect of care. The sensitive understanding of nurses and other health- and social-care practitioners in different areas of practice has helped us think more deeply about taking a lead in compassion. Our colleagues, throughout our careers in nursing, health visiting and education, have also been integral to our value system.

Following the writing of our first book, we found that each conference at which we spoke brought us into contact with others who feel as passionately as we do about compassion. That stimulated our thinking about how nurses, at all levels, can genuinely take a lead in influencing the quality of care in their practice areas.

We would like to thank Gillian Nineham and the whole team at Radcliffe Publishing for their unstinting support and encouragement throughout the marketing and conferences associated with our first book and the writing of this second book. We could not have hoped for a more supportive and friendly publisher.

We are also very grateful to Professor Sarah Kagan for her continuing invaluable support. Professor Kagan wrote the foreword for our first book and has written a highly insightful and emotive foreword to this second book.

We would particularly like to thank individuals and organisations who have contacted us and invited us to speak and write about compassion. These include Dee Cripps, Anne Barratt, the Janki Foundation for Global Health Care, the BBC Radio 4 Midweek programme team, Teresa Lynch, Joanna Goodrich and Jocelyn Cornwell of the King's Fund, the EMAP conference teams and various journals and magazines.

We were inspired by our attendance at the Inaugural and Second International Conferences on Compassionate Care in Edinburgh in June 2010 and 2011. The conferences were run by Edinburgh Napier University and NHS Lothian and brought together many people from throughout the world who were trying to generate a more compassionate caring environment for patients, clients and staff. It was clear that Stephen Smith, as lead nurse, and the rest of the Leadership in Compassionate Care programme team were highly committed to their work. It was also clear that students, such as Maria Carvalho and her colleagues, and ex-students were also engaged fully in the mindset of compassionate care.

From a personal point of view, we would like to thank all those who have been so encouraging about our writing. We would like to thank our parents, who have made us the people we are: Jack and Nancy Ephgrave and Ken and Monica Hale. In particular, we would like to thank the following people for their ongoing interest, encouragement and love: Irene, Amanda, Adrienne and Robert, as well as Dannii, Jessica, Ella, Louis, Chris, Jonathan, Amy and Anna.

Our special thanks to Alan Chambers and Malcolm Ryder, our ever-supportive husbands, who have been so encouraging and constructive in the help they have given in their different ways. They have been very much a part of this process, and are very proud of our achievements. Their unfailing support has helped us maintain our motivation throughout the writing of this book.

CHAPTER 1

Introduction: Excellence in compassionate nursing care – the importance of leadership

Overview of the chapter

Key theme one – the importance of compassion and caring in nursing

- Case study 1.1
- Compassion and caring in nursing – what is it?
- Thoughts for your practice
- Ongoing practice – discussion one
- Compassion and caring in nursing – why is it essential?
- Thoughts for your practice

Key theme two – compassion and caring in nursing: taking the lead

- Ongoing practice – discussion two
- Why do we need to take the lead on ensuring compassionate nursing?
- Thoughts for your practice
- Ongoing practice – discussion three
- What are the challenges to taking a lead on enhancing compassion in practice?
- Thoughts for your practice

Summary

References

OVERVIEW OF THE CHAPTER

Disillusioned, disempowered and angry is how nurses often feel about practice at the current time. They are trying to provide high-quality care and respond to the needs of patients, clients and carers as best they can. However, resources are very limited, shortages of staff and under-resourced teams are the norm and nurses feel that nobody is supporting them to enable them to provide caring, safe and effective nursing care. They feel they are doing the most they can possibly do within the resources available, but there is insufficient time to meet the complex needs of those in their care. They are constantly audited against targets that do not feel achievable or even beneficial to patients in their care. Everyone in their management hierarchy seems more concerned about outcomes, targets, number crunching and risk management than about patients. They do not feel valued or listened to and feel unable to take a lead in improving their service or in solving problems. They are criticised verbally and sometimes abused physically by patients, clients and their relatives, who are angry about the care that is, or is not, being provided. Sometimes the anger is justified, but nurses are angry too.

When will they be given enough staff to carry out their role?

When will they be able to finish their working day feeling that they have genuinely carried out their role as well as they would have wanted to?

When will managers actually understand the huge deficit of care and unmet needs that nurses face every day?

When will people start to acknowledge these issues and support them in the care they are trying to carry out?

When will they feel able to take a lead in solving some of the problems that they see affecting their service every day?

When will others stop delivering the final insult of criticising them for their lack of compassion? Don't they understand that wanting to deliver compassionate care is why they went into nursing in the first place?

Why can't people understand that nurses are frankly tired, burnt out, undervalued and criticised? When they feel so unappreciated, stressed and disempowered, it is very difficult for them to be as compassionate as they would like to be, or to create a more compassionate practice environment. 'Compassion can be defined in many ways, but its essence is a basic kindness, with a deep awareness of the suffering of oneself and of other living things, coupled with the wish and effort to relieve it' (Gilbert 2009, p. 11).

Patients, clients and nurses themselves would generally agree that kindness is a key attribute of nurses, and the one that underlies patients' perceptions of 'being cared about' as well as 'cared for'. The preceding quote highlights the importance of this innate kindness and the associated desire to relieve distress as being key to compassion. Nurses, more than most people, are in close contact with those needing relief from suffering, and although relief might not always be possible, a caring and kind attitude will undoubtedly help alleviate distress, while a lack of kindness will aggravate the distress.

However, in this incentive-driven and resource-constrained society in which we live and work, compassion and kindness might be seen as a weakness or a luxury when targets are more related to getting things done. Gilbert (2009) suggests that modern societies tend to overstimulate our incentive/resource-seeking and threat/self-protection systems to the detriment of our soothing/contentment system. This will inevitably lead to nurses – who essentially want to soothe and care for people – feeling stressed if they sense that this aspect of their role is not valued and that only the measurable quantitative outcomes of their practice are important.

According to Mooney (2009), nurses become burnt out with compassion overload and feel too stressed to be kind and compassionate when they are so busy. However, in our experience we have found that the opposite is true. Nurses tend to become stressed and distressed when they feel unable to be as compassionate as they would like to be, because of the sheer amount of work to be done. Firth-Cozens and Cornwell (2009), in their King's Fund report, agree with this perspective and say that 'if finance and productivity are perceived as being the only things that matter it can have profound negative effects on the way staff feel about the value placed on their work as care-givers. This makes it more difficult to cope with the inevitable emotional and psychological demands of the job' (p. 8).

They make a strong case for nurses having greater support in their early post-qualification years, to help them retain their compassion. Their report says (p. 5) that during training, nurses become less empathetic and more distanced from their patients, and that within 2 years of qualification their high-quality, patient-centred care becomes affected by frustration and burnout due to their ideals and values being thwarted.

According to Gilbert (2009), helping people to develop compassion is not always easy. Some people see compassion as a weakness or can be afraid of being drawn into the dreadfulness of someone's life experiences. In addition, compassionate care is potentially limited by insufficient resourcing. However, the nurse's attitude and the culture of the organisation are also essential components of the compassionate care environment. Therefore, modelling excellence in compassionate nursing care, through effective leadership, is essential for creating a compassionate environment.

This is not a book about leadership as such. At present, there are undoubtedly many constraints on nursing care that are detrimental to nurses and patients alike. This book, we hope, will help nurses to feel that they can take a lead in influencing nursing care to promote a compassionate care environment – wherever they work – an environment where uncompassionate care is not tolerated, where compassionate care is seen as the norm, and opportunities to develop compassionate care are encouraged and valued.

Breaking the style of leadership, from one based only on outcomes, throughput and efficiency to one in which compassion is focused around care and kindness, is essential to help others develop their compassionate approach to caring.

Staff are the most valued resource in any workplace, particularly in caring environments. If staff are not being treated with empathy, don't feel listened to, are not given choices where appropriate, are not empowered and helped to develop cultural competence, a compassionate environment and culture will not exist. Individuals who want to be compassionate will find themselves compromised. Therefore, nursing leaders, at all levels, need to foster this positive and compassionate care environment.

This chapter will focus on the importance of excellence in compassionate nursing care and how nurses can take a lead in creating a culture of caring. In the following chapters, case studies will be used to stimulate discussion and will be referred to in ongoing practice discussions throughout the chapter. Thoughts for practice will be drawn out to help readers further develop their own leadership practice in this important area of nursing care.

KEY THEME ONE – THE IMPORTANCE OF COMPASSION AND CARING IN NURSING

CASE STUDY 1.1

Sally was in the middle of a busy shift at the care home where she was the senior nurse. She knew that some members of her team felt disillusioned by caring for older people who did not appear to be always aware of what was going on around them, or even the care they were receiving. She had been very impressed with Rosa, who was a healthcare assistant and relatively new to the team, because she seemed to be very aware of the individual needs of each resident. Rosa seemed to genuinely enjoy the time she spent with the older people in her care. She would laugh and joke with them, and had said that she wanted to treat each resident as if they were her mother or her father.

Rosa had originally worked in the kitchen, but as she seemed to enjoy being with the residents so much, Sally had suggested that she become a healthcare assistant so that her skills with people could be used to maximum effect.

Sally knew that many of the members of her team did not share Rosa's personalised approach to care. For example, they would not ask residents whether they wanted sugar in their tea, or how many spoonfuls, because they assumed that residents would not know the difference. However, Rosa never took this approach. Sally saw Rosa bend down to talk to each resident and ask them how much sugar they wanted. She heard responses like 'No sugar for me, I'm sweet enough as I am' or 'Two sugars for me, I've got a sweet tooth'. Often these residents were not heard to speak at other times. Sally could see what a positive role model Rosa was to other more senior members of the team and resolved to make sure that Rosa knew what an excellent practitioner she was.

Compassion and caring in nursing – what is it?

This case study clearly demonstrates the value of personalised and patient- or client-centred care. Rosa was not prepared to take the quick approach by making assumptions – for example, about how residents liked their tea – but even so, her approach did not involve extra time.

Attitudes like this can seem very minor in the whole caring process, but can make such a difference between someone enjoying a cup of tea or not, due to them feeling respected and valued as an individual.

Rosa's situation is based on the experience of Maria Carvalho, who is about to qualify as a mental health nurse from Edinburgh Napier University. Maria used to be a kitchen assistant and then a healthcare assistant before she started her nursing programme. Maria is a very compassionate person by nature and in her nursing role, and was chosen to attend an inaugural conference on compassionate care.

Rosa's client-centred approach lies at the heart of compassionate care. Compassion is a highly complex concept and has different interpretations. For example, Frank (in Firth-Cozens and Cornwell 2009) sees compassion as involving an emotional response, both from the person giving the care as well as the person receiving it. He suggests that this 'goes beyond acts of basic care and is likely to involve generosity – giving a little more than you have to – kindness, and real dialogue' (p. 3). This real dialogue involves genuine interest and honesty, a recognition of difference rather than stereotyping and allows the practitioner to see the whole person behind the patient.

We do not believe that any care is 'basic', because in any intervention there is opportunity for assessment and advanced communication if the nurse's approach is holistic. However, the point Frank (2004) makes is that this complexity is inherent in compassionate care. Giving more than you absolutely have to, in any given situation, epitomises a compassionate approach to care, and often this does not involve more in the way of time and resources. Graber and Mitcham (2004), in an American study of hospital clinicians, sought to identify what specific actions, interventions and relationships were present in clinicians who were perceived as compassionate. They found that compassionate clinicians did not attempt to distance themselves from patients but developed warm and empathetic relationships with them, integrating mind and heart in their care while still retaining clinical objectivity.

NHS Lanarkshire in Scotland have embedded compassionate care in their practice, and they identify essential components of effective and compassionate relationships. They say that practitioners use their hands, heart and head and their practice is skilful, caring and knowledgeable. In order for this to be possible, support and direction is available through learning opportunities, feedback mechanisms and clear expectations (www.nhslanarkshire.org.uk).

Much that is written about compassion reflects the interpretations of different faiths, and much can be learnt from these spiritual perspectives. What underpins the compassionate approach demonstrated by Rosa has been fully developed by the Janki Foundation for Global Health Care, which has developed a Values in Healthcare pack (Janki Foundation for Global Health Care 2004). It emphasises the importance of the following values at all levels in healthcare practice:

➤ inner values
➤ peace
➤ positivity
➤ compassion
➤ cooperation
➤ valuing yourself
➤ spirituality in healthcare.

These values, or beliefs and principles, have an enormous effect on people's actions, behaviour and practice, whether they are in a caring role or not. Pendleton and King (2002) say that 'values are deeply held views that act as guiding principles for individuals and organisations. When they are declared and followed they are the basis of trust. When they are left unstated they are inferred from observable behaviour. When they are stated and not followed trust is broken' (p. 1352).

The Janki Foundation states that all these key personal attributes are central to providing excellent healthcare. They say that 'competence and compassion are the two most important aspects of healthcare. We would contend that compassion needs to be valued at least as much as competence in our work and in our education' (Janki Foundation for Global Health Care 2004, p. 193). Although competence is clearly paramount in healthcare, we do not believe that care is truly competent if it is not carried out with compassion.

The impact of an imbalance between competence and compassion is clearly demonstrated by Bridges *et al.* (2010), who focus on how older people can suffer from a 'diminished sense of significance' because of the perceived primacy of technical or medical care to the detriment of individuals' non-medical needs. According to Bridges *et al.* (2010), older patients and their relatives want staff in hospital to help them with:

➤ maintaining identity – 'see who I am' – patients want staff to know what is important to them, and relatives want staff to value what they know about the patient.
➤ creating community – 'connect with me' – a connected and two-way relationship with staff gives patients and relatives the reassurance that staff will care for them and meet their needs.
➤ sharing decision making – 'involve me' – patients and relatives want to understand what is happening, and to be given ongoing involvement in decision making.

In the case study, Rosa clearly saw who the individual person was, connected with them and involved them in the fundamental task of providing a cup of tea.

As Radcliffe (2010a) says, compassion is 'the thing that stops nursing being simply a list of acts aimed at well-being. Ask patients what makes the difference and they always say something that looks like compassion' (p. 23). Rosa's residents would have been in no doubt that they were in the presence of compassion.

In our book *Compassion and Caring in Nursing* (Chambers and Ryder 2009), we attempted to embrace these different perspectives on compassion and identified the following six key components of compassionate care:

➤ empathy and sensitivity
➤ dignity and respect
➤ listening and responding
➤ diversity and cultural competence
➤ choice and priorities
➤ empowerment and advocacy.

However compassion is interpreted, it is clear that care needs to be based on what patients and clients value in order for them to perceive it as person centred and caring. Focusing on how the recipient of the care might feel as a result of care can be challenging to busy nurses.

Is a compassionate and caring approach really essential in today's healthcare environment, or is it sufficient that care is simply safe and competent, when resources for healthcare are so limited?

In the next section, we will go back to our original case study and continue with our practice discussion. We will explore why we believe excellence in compassionate nursing care should be an essential feature of nursing practice.

THOUGHTS FOR YOUR PRACTICE

- How do you ensure that you have a person-centred approach to care?
- How do you ensure your practice is holistic and that you see the person, not the patient?
- Has this ever involved 'giving a little more than you have to'? If so, how did this make you feel?
- What values in healthcare underpin your practice? Do you find some values easier to make central to your practice than others? If so, why?
- How do you ensure that your patients, colleagues and students feel valued? How do you know this is the case?
- What approaches do you use to find out your patients' preferences?

ONGOING PRACTICE – DISCUSSION ONE

Sally was thinking about what was so special about Rosa's approach to residents in her care. Rosa was undoubtedly more interactive with people, and she certainly provoked more smiles and laughter. Residents had repeatedly told her how much better they felt when Rosa was on duty. So why was this? Rosa seemed not to spend any more time with individuals, but the quality of the time she did spend seemed to be far greater. She knew more about their lives, presumably because she had taken the time to ask questions, listen to the responses and remember them, so that she could build a picture of that person over her many contacts with them. She genuinely seemed to care about them as individuals, with different experiences, needs and preferences, and their faces tended to light up when she spoke to them. Sally knew that Rosa got through as much work in her shift as other nurses and healthcare assistants; in fact, often more so because she seemed to be able to work *with* residents to carry out the care from first greeting them. Other nurses seemed to spend a lot of time trying to persuade residents to 'cooperate', which seemed to cause a great deal of stress on both sides. Rosa, however, seemed to be able to use her personality and knowledge of the person concerned to carry out care that left people looking and feeling happier and more cared for. She seemed to instinctively know when someone was having a bad day or feeling miserable. At those times, she took the time to find out what was bothering them and still managed to complete what was needed in as short a time as possible. However, when the shift was less busy Sally could see Rosa talking to residents and doing small things for them that made a difference to their lives.

Compassion and caring in nursing – why is it essential?

Rosa's attitude towards those in her care clearly focused on the individuals themselves. It was essential to her perspective on nursing, and integral to her compassionate care. The importance of compassion is reflected in the Institute of Medicine's (2001) definition of patient-centred care, which emphasises key dimensions in relation to patient-centred care. These are:

➤ compassion, empathy and responsiveness to needs, values and expressed preferences
➤ coordination and integration
➤ information, communication and education
➤ physical comfort

➤ emotional support, relieving fear and anxiety
➤ involvement of family and friends.

Rosa was undoubtedly demonstrating compassion and empathy, and she valued residents' preferences. She was also concerned about physical and emotional comfort. Relatives and friends of the residents could tell that their loved ones were relaxed and cared for when Rosa was caring for them. Rosa also took time, when possible, to talk to visitors when they were there. She might not have been as involved with coordination, information and education, as that was Sally's responsibility, but her communication skills were clearly advanced. This example demonstrates why the Institute of Medicine's (2001) dimensions should be central to nursing care, in all nursing environments. Patients and clients know when they have been treated with compassion, even though they might find it difficult to define what this actually means.

However, in many areas of nursing practice, patients move through the system so fast that there is less opportunity for nurses to build even fleeting relationships. Meyer (2009) considers that this fast pace and the demands on nurses that take them away from direct nursing care are key factors that stand in the way of meaningful relationships.

Building relationships with residents in her care was a key component of Rosa's compassionate practice. A way of enhancing such relationships has been developed by Dewer *et al.* (2010) through the use of emotional touchpoints. These touchpoints are important events which are significant from the patient's perspective. Every individual builds up experiences of healthcare throughout their various interactions with health services and individual nurses. These experiences might be very diverse and many years apart, but they stay with the individual. If their experiences have been largely positive, then they might feel less anxious about needing care in the future. However, if they have been negative, these unresolved feelings will continue to have an impact on future experiences of healthcare. Such touchpoints are unique to each person; they comprise events that are particularly important to them, and they provoke unique emotions, whether positive or negative.

For example, someone who was disturbed while using the toilet and felt that their privacy and dignity had been violated might feel embarrassed, upset and angry. Conversely, someone who received sensitive help while using the toilet, through the use of appropriate and friendly communication, might feel that the nurse had made them feel less embarrassed, more respected and cared for. It is not necessarily the fact that something as private as going to the toilet has been witnessed that tends to cause distress; rather, it is how nurses carrying out this activity make the person feel.

This example shows how the emotional touchpoint of going to the toilet can elicit positive or negative feelings. Knowing how these experiences make people feel are key factors in delivering person-centred care. Dewar *et al.*'s (2010) work is part of the NHS Lothian and Napier University Leadership in Compassionate Care programme. Nurses appeared to feel much less threatened by receiving feedback about how patients felt in response to care that was given. This focus on patients' feelings meant that nurses did not feel blamed for how the care was carried out and responded less defensively. Better relationships with patients and their loved ones can develop as a result of them feeling part of enhancing the care given and the service provided. If people can discuss their negative or positive feelings about how something was carried out, learning for future practice developments can take place. It is essential that as nurses, we feel a sense of responsibility for the potential impact of our actions and interactions on a person's feelings about future healthcare.

This approach to quality enhancement is much less confrontational. By focusing on the positives as well as the lessons to be learnt, key learning is possible to enable nurses to take a lead in developing compassionate care in their practice environment. Nurses who are under pressure and feel undervalued need to hear positive feedback, otherwise they could feel criticised and defensive. Providing support in response to negative feedback and accepting positive feedback is key to nurses' self-esteem and morale, and it is the role of anyone taking on a leadership role to ensure that this is the case.

Meyer's (2009) point about the pace of nursing practice is a key reason why nurses often feel that they cannot provide the care that they want to. Clark (2010) discusses the dilemma of not knowing what a patient wants, even when there is sufficient time. For example, some people do not want to be rushed when they are having help with washing, while others just want care to be over as quickly as possible, particularly if this involves more intimate activities. In this case, using 'washing or bathing' as the emotional touchpoint would help to identify the different views of individual patients.

It is essential that nurses take the time to ensure that someone who has been independent until very recently but now needs help with fundamental care is treated with dignity and respect. A major life change such as this takes time to adapt to. As Burgess (2010) says, any of us would feel vulnerable and insecure and unused to having someone with us when we carry out personal care – people need sensitivity and time when these activities are being carried out. Not recognising or valuing this would be very easy in a busy environment and be the antithesis of the compassionate practice exemplified by Rosa in helping people to feel secure and valued.

Radcliffe (2010b) discusses the 'busyness' of nursing. He says that if nurses concentrate too much on the tasks of the day, it can be harmful to the nurses as well as those they care for. He feels that some nurses develop a 'walk of rage' – walking quickly, trying to get tasks achieved – to demonstrate how hard they are working and how much they are getting done. They do not value time that other nurses spend communicating with their patients, and their lack of work–life balance does not allow them to balance the emotional labour of nursing with other activities that might make them feel more fulfilled and valued. It is easy to see that in some nursing environments, this 'busy' approach is seen as the norm, and students and more junior members of the team might feel that they too have to adopt this approach in order to fit in. For nurses to take a lead in promoting compassionate practice, they need to appreciate the importance of having balance in their lives, and encouraging this in others. They also need to avoid acting as 'busy' role models, which others could emulate.

Williams *et al.* (2009) differentiate between 'pace' and 'complexity', particularly in relation to planning discharge of frail older people from acute hospital settings. This differentiation is transferable to all areas of nursing. Many nurses feel under pressure to concentrate on a fast pace of care and encourage a fast turnover of patients, so that their service appears as efficient as possible. This makes it particularly difficult to maintain a compassionate approach, and the fast turnover does not take into account the complexity of peoples' health and social circumstances.

An inappropriately fast discharge from hospital can result in a person being readmitted, because support networks are not in place to help them to cope in their home environment. This is not to the advantage of the hospital involved and it is deeply disempowering to the person concerned. There has been discussion of financial penalties for hospitals where readmissions take place within a short period of time. From the target- and resource-driven perspective, this is counterproductive, and the effect on the patient might be devastating to their future independence and well-being.

The issues we have discussed in this section clearly identify why compassionate care is essential and lies at the heart of person-centred practice.

We will take this discussion further in the next section by looking at what it means for all of us to take a lead to ensure that compassionate care is the central focus of practice.

THOUGHTS FOR YOUR PRACTICE

- How do you develop meaningful relationships with your patients?
- Think of an example from your practice of a patient's 'emotional touchpoint'. What did you learn from this, and how did this affect your future practice?
- How do ensure you meet the complex needs of your patients within the busy work environment?

KEY THEME TWO – COMPASSION AND CARING IN NURSING: TAKING THE LEAD

ONGOING PRACTICE – DISCUSSION TWO

Sally knew that Rosa was not very confident when it came to recognising her advanced skills in practice. Rosa wanted to be a nurse in the future, and Sally thought that she would be excellent in a nursing role and wanted to encourage her career development. Sally saw Rosa as a positive role model to others working in the care home, even though she had much less experience than some.

Rosa was not aware of how much difference she regularly made to residents' lives, and Sally felt that as the lead nurse of the home she had a responsibility to ensure that standards were as high as possible, that members of the team felt valued and that good practice was shared.

Sally spoke to Rosa at the start of her shift the following day. She made sure that residents' needs were being met, and then asked Rosa how she felt her skills were moving forward. When they talked in the office, which was quiet and private, Rosa was very quiet at first, but named various aspects of care that she felt that she could now do unsupervised. Sally agreed, and said that she was very pleased with how Rosa brought a fresh approach to the residential home. Rosa seemed surprised by this, and Sally went on to highlight several recent examples of excellent care that she had seen Rosa carry out. She said that she had noticed that Rosa always treated every resident as an individual, with their own needs and preferences. She said that she had noticed that the residents smiled more and laughed, and generally seemed more relaxed when she was around. Their loved ones often commented on how relieved they were to see their friend or relative feeling at home there. Sally explained it was all in the little things that she did, and the way she seemed to appear to really care for each individual, even when they were having a difficult day.

Rosa left the office feeling much more confident that she was able to work as a healthcare assistant and to carry out sensitive care. Sally had even said that she should apply for the next nursing programme, because she was sure that Rosa would be able to extend her skills and would make an excellent nurse. Rosa was so pleased that Sally felt this way and was very excited about the thought of becoming a nurse, and her mind was already full of ideas of how she would explain her passion for nursing on the application form.

Why do we need to take the lead on ensuring compassionate nursing?

Sally recognised Rosa's compassionate practice and clearly valued this as important. However, she also perceived herself as a leader, and as such recognised the importance of positive feedback and of her team members feeling valued. Many nurses spend their time feeling undervalued and in fact only get feedback when there is something negative to say. Being treated in an uncompassionate manner as a team member does not encourage a compassionate practice culture, where compassion is viewed as a key to caring practice.

It is essential that nurses recognise their role as leaders and act as positive role models, give appropriate and positive feedback and help others to feel valued members of the team. Fradd (2010) discusses the essential role that existing nurse leaders have in nurturing and encouraging the next generation of nurse leaders. Sally adopted this approach with Rosa. She recognised that Rosa was a very effective role model for compassionate care, and knew these skills needed to be nurtured. Fradd (2010) makes the point that increasing financial constraints mean that it is more important, not less, to identify and invest in those who will be able to take the nursing profession forward and innovate in practice with confidence.

Such valuing of clinical leadership is a central tenet in Lord Darzi's review (2009), which highlights nursing and nurse leadership roles as the key enablers in really transforming what happens for patients' experiences in a ward or the community.

Therefore, as Fradd (2010) says, 'nursing must grasp the opportunities to demonstrate the capability and capacity of nurses to lead' (p. 8). Yet how many nurses go through their day-to-day professional careers without feeling that they have a role to play in leadership? They are neither given opportunities to lead nor nurtured in their leadership role, and yet would have many good ideas for taking nursing practice forward. The emphasis on nurse leadership should allow these nurses to take a leadership role on different aspects of care, but managers must be prepared to actively seek their views, listen to their ideas and encourage their leadership development.

The Hay Group Growth Factor Inventory (www.haygroup.com) highlights the following factors in selecting staff for accelerated leadership development programmes:

➤ an eagerness and willingness to learn something new
➤ a breadth of perspective that enables the individual to take a wider view on issues
➤ an understanding of others
➤ personal maturity, which includes the ability to take feedback and use difficulties as a chance to learn.

Both Sally and Rosa could demonstrate these abilities in their different ways, and therefore should be nurtured as nurse leaders. However, Rosa is not yet a nurse, and Sally's sphere of influence is possibly not as great as it might be. She works in a care home and may have less opportunity to learn from others in the same role, or share good practice outside her immediate practice area. Therefore, their ability to be nurse leaders cannot be fully realised. However, Sally is using every opportunity she can to use her leadership skills.

Another reason why nurses must take the lead on ensuring excellence in compassionate nursing care relates to the changing role of nurses. Nursing has become increasingly task- and technically orientated, due to increased pressures to meet targets, with key personal-care roles being devolved to healthcare assistants. Therefore, student nurses could lack nursing role models in key areas of nursing care.

Healthcare assistants are often very experienced and can be excellent role models, but if student nurses value technical expertise over personal care, this could result in them not maintaining any kind of involvement or monitoring of important nursing care that is being carried out in their practice environment. This could lead to a lowering of standards, and as Allan and Smith (2010) point out, a failure to link education with practice in relation to personal care.

The direct relationship between leadership and quality of care is discussed by Hiscock and Shuldham (2008), who say that the expansion of the nurse role means that nurses are in 'a key position to influence and lead colleagues to improve patient care' (p. 900). If nurses are not involved in the fundamental care that is so key to their service, there is likely to be a negative impact on the quality of care received by patients. Sally was very aware that Rosa was a positive role model in relation to patient care. As a leader, Sally felt it was important to let Rosa know that her attitude, values and skills demonstrated sensitive nursing care.

Nurses often feel that if they are not a manager, they have no role in leading practice forward. Although they may be sensitive and effective practitioners themselves, they might not feel that they should have a role in influencing the care given by others.

This can result from a lack of understanding about the difference between leadership and management. Kotter (2001) says that management is about 'order and consistency', whereas leadership is about 'coping with change' (p. 86). He identifies four different areas of activities and states how management and leadership are both key components of these activities, although the perspectives and tasks are different. These different activities are represented in Table 1.1.

TABLE 1.1 Differences between management and leadership: a representation of Kotter's activities (Kotter 2001)

	MANAGEMENT	LEADERSHIP
CREATING AGENDA	Planning and budgeting	Setting a direction
DEVELOPING HUMAN RESOURCES	Organising and staffing	Aligning people
EXECUTION	Controlling and problem solving	Motivating people
OUTCOMES	Producing a degree of predictability	Promoting positive change strategies

Kotter (2001) makes the point that in times of great change, greater leadership is needed. Healthcare today is so multidimensional, multicultural and multifaceted that response to change is required very quickly. As nurses are at the forefront of most of these changes, they need to have excellent leadership skills to guide the service forward in a manner that ensures that providing compassionate care remains central.

Taking a lead in relation to compassionate care can be a challenge for nurses today. Resource constraints mean that nurses are overworked, stressed and demotivated. When morale is poor, people become defensive. Nurses can feel that their whole professional identity is being challenged when there are calls for greater compassion in nursing care. Because 'being compassionate' was their main impetus for becoming a nurse, they do not always feel positive about taking a lead role to ensure that compassion is central to nursing practice. Instead, they may feel defensive and concentrate on the lack of resources that makes practice so difficult for them. However, if nurses do not take a lead on compassion and on how the patient experience can be enhanced, who will?

When care is not optimal, sensitivity is needed to ensure that colleagues are not alienated and that beleaguered practitioners do not feel scapegoated, but instead feel positive about finding new ways to create a caring environment in an under-resourced service.

If nurses are to be leaders in practice, and in compassionate care, they need to be emotionally intelligent. Goleman (2002) states that emotional intelligence incorporates personal competence, in the form of self-awareness and self-management, and social competence, in the form of social awareness and relationship management. This will be discussed in later chapters in relation to individual nurse attitude and creating a practice culture that is sensitive and compassionate. Marques (2007) says that in terms of leadership, emotional intelligence and passion are interconnected. She makes the point that if a leader is not passionate about their role, then it might be better if they were not a leader at all. Nurses who are in a management role might have lost their passion for their leadership role, but there are nurses who have also lost their passion for nursing in its entirety.

We have said that all nurses can be leaders in some way. However, if nurses lack passion for their role and cannot identify with the needs of their patients, they are certainly in no position to lead the service forward. If nurse managers have lost the passion for management (maybe because they miss their clinical role), or never had it in the first place, then again they cannot be compassionate to the stresses of those that they manage. When listening to discussions of nurses and managers in practice. One gets the impression that this lack of passion is more common than many of us would like to think. For the service to adapt to the many changes that are part of healthcare today, nurses need to rediscover their passion for nursing, or their management role, and develop greater passion for leadership and enhancing practice.

Marques (2007) says that without emotional intelligence, a leader cannot relate to the hidden messages behind what someone is saying, or the things that are not being said. This occurs with leaders who are so stressed themselves that they cannot identify unhealthy stress levels in their colleagues, or understand that another change would be a step too far at the moment. Insensitive leadership of this sort only adds to the stress that a nurse might already be feeling about their practice role, and causes them to feel more undervalued and misunderstood. The only option for the nurse at this point may be to go off sick, which is counterproductive to a service that can ill afford higher absence levels when it is already under-resourced. It is also counterproductive to the nurse, who might return to work with no better coping strategies and feeling just as desperate as before, and can lead to ongoing poor mental health with frequent times of sickness.

Nurse leaders also need to be able to deal with conflict, ensure their emotional responses are appropriate and handle emotions and relationships with others (Goleman 1998). The ability to problem solve and understand emotions and respond appropriately is a key component of leadership (Mayer *et al.* 1999). Yet there is much anecdotal evidence of nurse managers not treating colleagues with respect, expressing inappropriate emotions and being unable to understand the emotional needs of others, or being unable to problem-solve or to predict or deal with conflict. This can only lead to greater problems in the workplace, and when practice is even more stressful and staffing levels are even lower, can make the difference between a safe and effective service and an unsafe one. In the previous practice discussion, we noted that Sally was a compassionate leader because she understood that Rosa needed to feel valued and respected. We would argue that compassionate leadership is not optional but is an integral part of good practice. Positive feedback on Rosa's relationships with residents helped Rosa to feel positive about her practice, and Sally's confidence in Rosa's ability to be a nurse would have meant a great deal. Compassionate leadership is more likely to lead to more compassionate practice.

Marques (2007) makes a strong case for leaders to be innovative, to be competent in their role, to have technical expertise if necessary and to persevere in difficult circumstances. We agree that innovation is a necessity in times of constant change. In addition, the ability of an individual to persevere when their role is difficult, without becoming openly stressed and stressful to work with, is essential to a positive work environment. The final attribute of a good leader, according to Marques (2007), is charisma. We also see this as essential because charismatic leaders can communicate well and draw out the positives, taking others with them when they have innovative ideas.

Marques (2007) sums up her interesting paper on the connection between emotional intelligence and passion in relation to leadership by saying that charisma and love for both the work and the progress to be made, and for the people and the environment, are integral to good leadership. The underlying communication that encapsulates all these concepts allows this to be passed on to others. We would argue that the reason most people come into nursing in the first place is because of their good communication skills, passion for their role, emotional intelligence and love for the work and the people they care for, so all nurses should be naturally good leaders. If any of these elements have diminished over the years, or need to be rediscovered, then now is the time for that to happen. As we have said, great change and challenging times need great leaders. Nursing has always had strong leadership, but perhaps now all nurses should see themselves as leaders and work towards making practice the best it can be, within available resources.

Resources are often perceived as being a key challenge for compassionate care. In the next section, we will discuss other challenges to enhancing excellence in compassionate nursing care.

THOUGHTS FOR YOUR PRACTICE

- Are there nurses who you feel are excellent role models for you in terms of being a leader of nursing?
- How could you benefit from their approaches and expertise as leaders?
- Do you feel that you are in a position to enhance the patient experience of care? If so, how would you do this? If not, what is standing in your way?
- What can you do to take a lead in moving practice forward in your own practice environment?
- How do you think you could take a lead in ensuring that high-quality care is the norm in your practice area? How can you ensure that all members of the team carry out care to this high standard?
- How can you help others to cope with the challenge of change?
- How can you respond to the defensiveness of others who feel criticised for lower standards of care than they would want to give?
- Do you still feel passionate about your role? How can you help others to rediscover their passion for nursing?

ONGOING PRACTICE – DISCUSSION THREE

Sally was so impressed with Rosa's approach to residents in her care that she wanted other carers working in the home to be aware of how Rosa approached different tasks. She did not want them to feel criticised or defensive about what they had been doing, just to think about different ways of working.

So at the next handover meeting, Sally said that she really wanted to celebrate the excellent care she saw within the home. She asked the carers to think about the things they did in their day-to-day work that made a positive difference to residents' lives, so that they could discuss them at the next meeting.

When the carers came to the meeting, they were reticent to talk about their own practice, including Rosa. Those whom Sally knew to be excellent carers did not see their actions as significant: they thought it was how everyone would be. She knew, however, that this was not the case and that others were not all as caring or as empathetic.

Sally carried on with the discussion and pointed out examples of good care that she had seen. She used examples from everyone's practice, not just Rosa's. With those who appeared more rushed, or who did not communicate quite so easily, she used positive examples from when this had not been the case. She could see people begin to open up and start to smile, and soon they all seemed to be more positive than they had been at the start of the meeting.

She asked them if they wanted to use the whiteboard in the office to highlight others' good practice when they saw it, and they seemed to think this was a good idea. A week later, the board was full of examples and Sally could tell that the atmosphere among the carers was more positive and that they communicated much more positively with other carers and residents too.

What are the challenges to taking a lead on enhancing compassion in practice?

Sally clearly had a passion for nursing, good practice and her leadership role, as discussed in the previous section. She was skilled at creating a positive environment where good practice was shared and where people felt valued.

One approach designed to strengthen a positive environment of care is the Senses Framework (Nolan *et al.* 2006). Initially this was designed to help students who would be working with older people to feel positive about their practice area. The framework focused around students feeling:

➤ a sense of security – it was safe to explore the nursing role
➤ a sense of belonging – they were a member of the ward team
➤ a sense of continuity – links between theory and practice and supported by a mentor
➤ a sense of purpose – their own learning needs were prioritised by others
➤ a sense of achievement – that they could meet their learning objectives
➤ a sense of significance – they could contribute in a way that mattered.

As a result, students felt valued and more positive about their practice. The approach has been now been broadened and used in other practice areas, moving away from person-centred care, which could be perceived as a narrow view of care, towards relationship-centred care. The individual behind the condition is perceived as being central to the care process and the focus is on 'care' not merely 'cure'. This holistic framework recognises that people communicate and have relationships with others in a wider context. It reflects the balance between the needs of patients, families, communities and practitioners, and all groups are perceived as having equal value, status and significance.

Sally in her own way was adopting this positive and relational approach to practice, and staff in the care home would have felt a sense of security in sharing their practice ideas, as well as a sense of belonging, continuity, purpose, achievement and significance. However, the challenges for Sally were to ensure that all members of the team felt positive about their practice, and having sufficient time to create the right environment for this discussion – not always easy to achieve in practice, despite nurses having the advanced communication skills, emotional intelligence and sensitivity that Sally clearly possessed.

The Senses Framework (Nolan *et al.* 2006) emphasises the need to move away from the concept of purely curing towards the concept of caring. This also links with the need to 'care about' and not merely 'care for' people and the need to focus on relationship-based rather than task-orientated care (Chambers and Ryder 2009, Maben *et al.* 2010, Meyer 2009, de Raeve 2002). However, when time is short it can be easier to focus on technical and medical tasks.

The importance of being 'cared about' was emotionally described by Professor Kieran Sweeney, who was only 57 years old when he was diagnosed with a malignant mesothelioma. As a doctor who was used to treating people who were ill, but who had always been well himself, he expresses very clearly the shock and distress of being 'dispatched to the kingdom of the sick permanently and irretrievably' (Sweeney *et al.* 2009, p. 511). He says that he was treated with technical competence, but makes the point that healthcare professionals tended to keep the locus of control, and therefore acted in a directional or transactional manner, rather than in a relational way that allowed him to feel cared about. He said, 'What I have always feared in illness was anonymity, being packaged, losing control, not being able to say "this is who I am." In the end, one is left alone, here, in the kingdom of the sick' (Sweeney *et al.* 2009, p. 512).

However short time may be, it is essential that nurses relate to the person behind the patient, and respect their fears and concerns when providing care. Sometimes simply carrying out a task is all that is required, or all that there is time for. However, at other times relationship-based care is possible and very much needed. Professor Sweeney needed this sort of care to overcome his feelings of being alone and uncared for, and so do all people in our care. Goodrich (2009) differentiates between high and low levels of transactional care, where things are either efficient but impersonal or unpleasant and inefficient. In relational care, everything works when levels are high, whereas things are warm but chaotic if levels are low. Therefore, the most compassionate and effective care occurs where there are high levels of both transactional and relational aspects of care (*see* Figure 1.1 below).

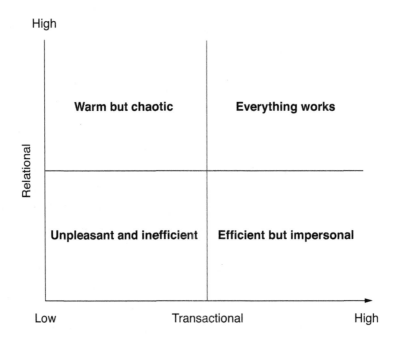

FIGURE 1.1 Transactional and relational aspects of care (Goodrich 2009)

The importance of these are highlighted by Sean Brophy in his paper on compassion in healthcare. Brophy (2010) talks about his care towards the end of his life and compares the approaches of five different nurses who were called to an elderly man in a neighbouring bed, whose intravenous line kept disconnecting. The first four nurses just reconnected the cannula and went away, leaving the man ever more agitated as it disconnected again and again. The fifth nurse, however, said to him that she would take care of him; she secured the drip with tape and said kindly that it was safe to go to sleep now – she acted with compassion. Brophy said that at the time there was no shortage of nurses on duty; the difference was in the compassionate care shown by that one nurse.

The challenge of retaining the 'art' of nursing as well as the 'science' is faced by many nurses today. Brophy (2010) agrees with the quote from Hawkins that 'medicine is not a science; medicine is an art for which medical science is a tool' (Hawkins 2002, cited in Brophy 2010, p. 21). This is equally true of nursing; the art of medicine and nursing lies in the holistic, relationship-based, creative and unique approaches that healthcare professionals use in their interactions with patients and clients. However, if we reduce nursing to a set of tasks that can be quantified and measured, this will undermine the therapeutic value of what we do, and how people feel as a result of our care.

Healthcare today is a business, and as such there have to be measurable parameters as indicators of success. Quality indicators are used as a measure of success, but is it really quality of care that is being measured, or simply the number of quantifiable tasks that have been carried out? Maben *et al.* (2010) describe how in these audit-driven times, second-order (measurable) activities are valued more highly than first-order (intimate relationship-based) activities. Therefore, 'the art of caring is both invisible and subordinated' (Maben *et al.* 2010, p. 11). They say that the emphasis on targets and clinical care can have a strong negative impact on the importance of the patient experience.

This can be why 'being seen to be busy' is a major priority for some nurses. Brophy (2010) cites Menzies (1960) term of 'legitimate gait' where nurses who want to avoid engagement with a patient walk fast and avoid all eye contact, or avoid contact with patients when possible by congregating around the nurses' station. Sweeney *et al.* (2009) also talk about the avoidance of eye contact and say how distressing this can be to a patient. Radcliffe (2010b) makes the point that some nurses justify themselves to others and protect themselves from criticism by walking fast as a way of showing how hard they are working.

So are nurses concentrating on targets and tasks that are easily measurable purely in order to meet what is required of them by senior management, or is there another reason for this distancing from a patient's distress?

Much has been written about the emotional labour of nursing and of emotional distress and burnout. Meyer (2009) says that nurses could be distancing themselves from patients and concentrating on specific tasks as a psychological defence against the pain they might feel if they empathised too strongly with those in distress. Maben *et al.* (2010) say that 'really relating to patients takes courage, humility and compassion' (p. 11) and that nurses need constant renewal, recognition and support from colleagues and managers to be able to carry on giving at this level. However, the nurses we have spoken to are not compassion fatigued, but deeply distressed by being too busy to give the empathetic and compassionate care they would like to provide. Radcliffe (2010b) says that 'unmanaged, unending commitment to the tasks of the day becomes corrosive for many healthcare workers' and thinks that 'it makes some people unhappy, some people unwell and some people not very good at their jobs' (p. 26).

Why do nurses lose the empathy and compassion that was so evident when they came into nursing? Mooney (2009) draws from the King's Fund report (Firth-Cozens and Cornwell 2009), which says that nurses lose compassion, or experience some level of burnout, in the first 2 years of practice. West (2010) discusses how nurses can become desensitised to poor care, and how lack of compassion can become the norm in some practice areas. So how does this impact on morale, staff turnover and role modelling for students and more junior members of the team? Managers and leaders have a strong role to play in providing support to nurses who are at risk of reducing their expression of care for others, whether they be patients, clients, colleagues or their managers. As Radcliffe (2010c) says, 'something happens to nurses who perform badly. Something disables them. It may be anything from burnout to breakdown, from mismanagement to disinvestment. A lack of professional sustenance or no supervision. But nurses do not nurse badly for no reason' (p. 24).

If quantifiable outcomes are so important in today's healthcare environment, how do we measure compassion, and is it possible to even try? From 2010, as part of their entry criteria, universities in Wales will be assessing potential students' ability to demonstrate compassion. Students will be asked for a character statement and assessed at interview on their understanding of caring. They will also be assessed in practice placement for attitudinal skills such as responsiveness to feedback and a caring disposition. The patient perspective will need to be included in this assessment too, because although a mentor can observe caring gestures and words, only the patient or client can measure whether it feels caring to them. Firth-Cozens and Cornwell (2009) in the King's Fund Point-of-Care programme say that the patient experience is key to assessing the presence or absence of compassion, because it needs to be felt by both the carer and the patient. When it comes to compassion, Radcliffe (2010a) says, 'Compassion is no harder to measure than rain. Is there rain? Stand outside and you'll know. Is there compassion? Be around it, you'll know' (p. 23).

The King's Fund report (Firth-Cozens and Cornwell 2009) identifies various factors that inhibit compassion, namely (i) the values instilled in clinical training – hopefully these are now more caring orientated than they were some years ago, (ii) a fear of distress and dying, and of stress, depression and overload, which we have discussed already, and (iii) the wider hospital environment with organisational structures that are inflexible and do not focus on the individual. A nurse leader can help to alleviate these factors by ensuring that there is a focus on teaching compassion, by providing opportunities to get closer to patients, by role modelling of caring nursing and by providing positive and constructive feedback to nurses in their practice areas. Westwood (2010) lists several ways in which nurses can encourage compassionate care:

➤ Be clear about what compassion means to you.
➤ Act with compassion whether you feel like it or not.
➤ Find others who want to change things and form a team, being specific about what you want to see change.
➤ Be compassionate to yourself to recharge your batteries.
➤ Give positive feedback to others and thank them, whatever grade you are, even if you are not getting that kind of feedback yourself.
➤ Get help and support if you are struggling.

If nurses can take a lead by adopting these strategies, they will make a difference to patients' experience.

The King's Fund report (Firth-Cozens and Cornwell 2009) identified that patients' experience was influenced by the following:

➤ the patient and family
➤ individual staff members
➤ the team, unit and department
➤ the hospital
➤ the wider healthcare system.

Strong nurse leaders at all levels and in all care environments are needed to influence these factors. Masterson and Gough (2009, 2010) say how important it is for leaders to be flexible and able to deal with ambiguity and uncertainty in order to influence the wider healthcare environments in which they work. They also need to be trustworthy, have advanced communication skills and have high levels of self-awareness about their own strengths and limitations, their emotional intelligence and their ability to communicate a vision and motivate others.

These strong nurse leaders need to challenge poor care and set and maintain standards, and should be at all levels in the organisation. As Radcliffe (2009) says 'We should hand the job back to nurses. Not the defensive ones. Not the tired ones. Not even the powerful ones. No, we should give it to the 'ordinary' nurses – the nurses who burn with anger when they hear of patients left to lie in wet beds' (p. 34).

THOUGHTS FOR YOUR PRACTICE

- What helps you, your students and colleagues to feel positive about practice? Can you think of other ways to strengthen this?
- How do you ensure you 'care about' your patients and not just 'care for' them?
- How do you ensure that your practice is as relationship based as possible when you are carrying out nursing tasks?
- Have you ever used being 'busy' to avoid building relationships with patients or clients? If so, do you think this was always justified? How do you think the patient felt as a result?
- Do you feel that you sometimes have not got the emotional reserves to really identify with patients in distress? If so, what would help you with this?
- Do you feel stressed by not being able to give adequate emotional care to patients? Is there anything that would help you with this?
- How do you ensure your practice, and that of others, is a balance between quality of care and measurable outcomes?

SUMMARY

In this chapter, we have focused on the difficulties faced by highly committed nurses working in complex healthcare environments. Nurses want to maintain a compassionate approach to patients and clients at all times, but this can sometimes be very difficult.

The chapter has discussed the importance of ensuring excellence in compassionate nursing care, particularly in today's healthcare environment. It is essential for patients and clients, but also for nurses, who can find it difficult to accept the fact that they are not always able to give people the time that they need.

Every nurse, whatever their position, has a leadership role in taking nursing practice forward, and ensuring that compassionate care remains at the heart of practice.

The challenges are undeniable, and in our previous book (Chambers and Ryder 2009) we noted that they cluster around three main areas that influence practice. These are:

➤ resourcing issues
➤ the culture of the organisation
➤ nurses' attitudes.

We will use these three areas as the focus for our next three chapters and hope our discussions will help nurses to feel that they really can make a difference, and encourage them to take a lead in ensuring that care is compassionate in their own practice environments.

REFERENCES

Allan H, Smith P. It is the education system that leads students to reject basic care. *Nurs Times.* 2010; **106**(1): 9.

Bridges J, Flatley M, Meyer J. Older people's and relatives' experiences in acute care settings: systematic review and synthesis of qualitative studies. *Int J Nurs Stud.* 2010; **47**(1): 89–107.

Brophy S. Compassion in healthcare: a patient's perspective. *NHS Lothian and Edinburgh Napier University Inaugural International Conference on Compassionate Care.* 2010 Jun 9–11; Edinburgh.

Burgess J. I've seen real dignity in care, and know what it requires. *Nurs Times.* 2010; **106**(19): 23.

Chambers C, Ryder E. *Compassion and Caring in Nursing.* Oxford: Radcliffe Publishing; 2009.

Clark J. Defining the concept of dignity and developing a model to promote its use in practice. *Nurs Times.* 2010; **106**(20): 16–19.

Darzi A. *High Quality Care for All: our journey so far.* London: Department of Health; 2009.

de Raeve L. Trust and trustworthiness in nurse–patient relationships. *Nurs Philos.* 2002; **3**(2): 152–62.

Dewar B, Mackay R, Smith S, *et al.* Use of emotional touchpoints as a method of tapping into the experience of receiving compassionate care in a hospital setting. *J Res Nurs.* 2010; **15**(1): 29–41.

Fradd E. Positive action: it is surprising the nursing profession has not collectively responded to the leadership challenge. *Nurs Times.* 2010; **106**(8): 8–9.

Frank A. The renewal of generosity; illness, medicine and how to live. 2004. In: Firth-Cozens J, Cornwell J. *The Point of Care: enabling compassionate care in acute hospital settings.* London: King's Fund; 2009.

Firth-Cozens J, Cornwell J. *The Point of Care: enabling compassionate care in acute hospital settings.* London: King's Fund; 2009.

Gilbert P. *The Compassionate Mind.* London: Constable and Robinson; 2009.

Goleman D. Boyatzis R, McKee A. *The New Leaders: transforming the art of leadership into the science of results.* London: Sphere; 2002.

Goleman D. The emotionally competent leader. *Healthc Forum J.* 1998; **41**(2): 36–8.

Goodrich J. Transactional and relational aspects of care. In: Understanding the Patient Experience of Care. *Second Annual Nursing Times Nursing Quality Conference Delivering High Quality Nursing Care.* 2009 Nov 18; London.

Graber DR, Mitcham MD. Compassionate clinicians; take patient care beyond the ordinary. *Holist Nurs Pract.* 2004; **18**(2): 87–94.

Hawkins D. Power vs. force: the hidden determinants of human behaviour. 2002. In: Brophy S. Compassion in Healthcare: a patient's perspective. *NHS Lothian and Edinburgh Napier University Inaugural International Conference on Compassionate Care.* 2010 Jun 9–11; Edinburgh.

Hay Group. *Growth Factor Inventory (GFI).* Available at: www.haygroup.com/leader shipandtalentondemand/ourproducts/item_details.aspx?itemid=91&type=2&t=2 (accessed 13 January 2012).

Hiscock M, Shuldham C. Patient centred leadership in practice. *J Nurs Manag.* 2008; **16**(8): 900–4.

Institute of Medicine. To err is human: building a safer health system. 2001. In: Goodrich J, Cornwell J. *Seeing the Person in the Patient.* London: King's Fund; 2008.

Janki Foundation for Global Health Care. *Values in Healthcare: a spiritual approach.* London: Janki Foundation for Global Health Care; 2004.

Kotter J. What leaders really do. *Harvard Business Review.* 2001 Dec 1. pp. 85–96.

Maben J, Cornwell J, Sweeney K. In praise of compassion. *J Res Nurs.* 2010; **15**(1): 9–13.

Marques JF. Leadership: emotional intelligence, passion and . . . what else? *J Manag Dev.* 2007; **26**(7): 644–51.

Masterson A, Gough P. On how to design a leadership programme to boost quality. *Nurs Times.* 2009; **105**(24): 27.

Masterson A, Gough P. Adaptable leaders are crucial to the new NHS. *Nurs Times.* 2010; **106**(34): 23.

Mayer J, Caruso D, Salovey P. Emotional intelligence meets traditional standards for an intelligence. *Intelligence.* 2000; **27**(4): 267–98.

Menzies I. A case study in the functioning of social systems as a defence against anxiety. *Hum Relat.* 1960; **13**: 95–121.

Meyer J. Promoting dignity, respect and compassionate care. *J Res Nurs.* 2009; **15**(1): 69–73.

Mooney H. Compassion is early casualty of nurse frustration and burnout. *Nurs Times.* 2009; **105**(15): 2.

Nolan M, Brown J, Davies S, *et al. The Senses Framework: improving care for older people through a relationship-centred approach.* Sheffield: University of Sheffield; 2006.

Pendleton D, King J. Values and leadership. *BMJ.* 2002; **325**(7376): 1352–5.

Radcliffe M. Compassion is no harder to measure than rain. *Nurs Times*. 2010a; **106**(17): 23.

Radcliffe M. The good, the bad, and the ridiculously busy. *Nurs Times*. 2010b; **106**(28): 26.

Radcliffe M. Why understand if you can just point the finger? *Nurs Times*. 2010c; **106**(25): 24.

Radcliffe M. The job of basic care should be handed back to nurses. *Nurs Times*. 2009; **105**(35): 34.

Sweeney K, Toy L, Cornwell J. A patient's journey: mesothelioma. *BMJ*. 2009; **339**(b2862): 511–14.

West D. Nurses at risk of compassion fatigue. *Nurs Times*. 2010; **106**(9): 3.

Westwood C. Nursing with compassion: what can you do? Available at: www.nursing times.net/nursing-with-compassion-what-can-you-do/5014361.article (accessed 15 October 2010).

Williams S, Nolan M, Keady J. Relational practice as the key to ensuring quality care for frail older people: discharge planning as a case example. *Quality in Ageing and Older Adults*. 2009; **10**(3): 44–55.

www.nhslanarkshire.org.uk/boards/Archive/2009BoardPapers/Documents/May%20 2009/Caring%20and%20Compassionate%20Practice%20Guide%20-%20May%20 2009%20Board.pdf

CHAPTER 2

Compassionate care – the challenge of resourcing

Overview of the chapter

Key theme one – resources for compassionate care

- Case study 2.1
- What is the relationship between resourcing and providing compassionate care?
- Thoughts for your practice
- Ongoing practice – discussion one
- How could the challenge of resourcing potentially have a negative impact on our relationship with patients and clients?
- Thoughts for your practice

Key theme two – taking the lead on influencing resourcing

- Ongoing practice – discussion two
- What is our role in taking this lead?
- Thoughts for your practice
- Ongoing practice – discussion three
- How can we take a lead in keeping compassionate care at the heart of nursing, despite resource constraints?
- Thoughts for your practice

Summary

References

OVERVIEW OF THE CHAPTER

We have chosen to discuss resourcing issues as the first challenge facing those wanting to taking a lead on ensuring excellence in compassionate nursing care, because it is such an important area of concern. Today's healthcare environment is so financially constrained that nurses feel deeply concerned about the care that they are unable to give, and the immense pressures on their time. When the care is not at an optimal level, they are the ones who are on the receiving end of critical comments from patients, friends and family, as well as other nurses and healthcare professionals. They usually know when they have not been able to achieve a 'good enough' service, let alone excellent levels of care. They have, however, done the best they could within the staffing and resources available.

When people feel vulnerable or unwell, they become anxious, and that anxiety can be expressed as anger. Bradshaw (1972), in his seminal text, discussed different concepts of needs. The normative needs are those that exist from a professional's perspective. From a nurse's point of view, these would, at times, primarily relate to a patient's safety, because this is the greatest priority. So in an acute situation, a patient who was at risk of life-threatening deterioration would have the highest priority and another patient's toileting need would be secondary. In a less acute situation, someone who was experiencing great distress would have higher priority than others who are waiting. The nurse is constantly balancing competing comparative needs and making prioritising decisions. Meanwhile, waiting patients or their loved ones could be experiencing feelings of anxiety, pain, discomfort, isolation or vulnerability, which they see as their priority, but these may not be perceived as important to the nurse, or the nurse might not be able to spend enough time with them to really understand what is important to them. Their needs might therefore not be manifested to the nurse as feelings, but may be expressed as verbal or physical anger, which would increase the nurse's stress levels even more.

It is important that the needs of all concerned are prioritised at some point, but this cannot always be done as promptly as the patient or client feels that it should be. One of the problems here is the length of the nursing 'minute'; when a nurse says that they will be back in a 'minute', it is not necessarily an accurate representation of the elapsed time because something more urgent might have taken place during that 'minute'. Some nurses try to be more precise about when they hope to return, and the language they use to express this. Even when saying that you cannot deal with something immediately, it is possible to be compassionate in what you say and how you say it to the person on the receiving end. Yet many patients comment that nurses always seem to be in a rush, avoid eye contact and seem to want to get away as quickly as possible, even when they are attending a patient. This is counterproductive to both the nurse and the patient because both would feel much better if care had been carried out in a compassionate manner. It doesn't necessarily take more time to provide genuine, compassionate and person-centred care.

Although caring tasks take time to carry out, the time might not require total involvement of the nurse. For example, blood pressure can be measured with the nurse either being actively engaged with the patient or working more as a technician. Other assessment tools can involve so much documentation that the process of asking the questions can remove all compassion from the assessment. An example of this was a student nurse who was trying to record the family history with a new mother in the community. Due to her inexperience, she focused exclusively on the record sheet and failed to be aware of the mother's distress when asked whether her mother was alive and well. The client replied that her mother had died only a few months before. She was visibly still very much in the acute stage of bereavement, and yet the student nurse carried on asking questions, without looking up or acknowledging the pain in the client's voice. However, it is not only inexperienced nurses who can miss the opportunity to engage with the patient; a nurse giving antibiotics to a patient who had just returned from theatre spent the time looking out the window rather than assessing the patient's health status or communicating with them.

Nurses are not mere technicians. They have skills of intuition and assessment (the 'art' of nursing) that are much better than the technology they use, but if they allow technology to dominate and be a hindrance to assessment and communication, a great deal of information will be lost. As Sills (2010) says, 'Without interaction nurses do not have the full picture – it is not a machine that will develop intuitive skills' (p. 13). Nurses' instinct and intuition are skills developed through years of observation, listening and communicating with patients and clients and have saved many a patient from deterioration and even death. Loss of these skills would be the loss of the true expertise of nursing and without them we would become mere automatons.

This chapter focuses on the challenge of resourcing issues in relation to taking a lead in compassion, using a case study that will be developed through the chapter as ongoing practice discussions. We consider the importance of resourcing for compassionate care, the potential resources required – and why they are central to people for whom we care, and finally we focus on taking the lead on influencing resourcing, in terms of what role nurses can play and how we can lead change in relation to maintaining a compassionate approach despite resource constraints.

KEY THEME ONE – RESOURCES FOR COMPASSIONATE CARE

CASE STUDY 2.1

Swapna had always felt so comfortable with the Community Children's Nursing Team. She knew that she was no longer a child and needed to have her care managed by nurses who cared for adults, but it felt like such an alien world to her. She knew who everyone was and how the systems worked in children's services, whereas now she felt out of control. It was bad enough having cystic fibrosis in the first place. It limited her life so much, but she had always been determined that it would not define who she was. She knew that there did not seem to be as many services in the adult team and she did not really know how her care needs could be met in this new world. The children's nursing team had spent time preparing her for the transition, but since moving from their care nothing had seemed to go right – she had been admitted to hospital three times with symptoms that would previously have been managed at home. Her case manager in the new team was a nurse called Vikas. Vikas had rung her earlier that day, following her discharge from hospital yesterday, and had asked to come to see her in his role as community matron. She did not really know what community matrons did, and with a title such as matron she was surprised any of them were male. Although Vikas had introduced himself on the phone, she still did not know what to expect from this visit, but she did know that she did not want to keep having emergency admissions to hospital.

What is the relationship between resourcing and providing compassionate care?

Swapna had clearly felt very reassured by the care she received throughout her childhood years, but was now considered an adult by the care services, as well as by herself. She wanted to take control of her life, and of her health and illness, and did not want to remain dependent on others. She wanted to plan her life and could not do so when her illness was so unpredictable.

Vikas had never met Swapna and did not know what her concerns or her priorities were. He wanted to start to build his relationship with her by introducing himself and his role, but his main priority for the visit was to try to see how Swapna viewed her illness, how it impacted on her life and what was important to her. Stevenson (2002), in his Australian paper, highlights how important it is for the patient to feel that care is centred on them. Patients are more likely to feel satisfied with their care, and there are likely to be fewer referrals, investigations and malpractice complaints, and more positive outcomes as a result. In addition, there is greater concordance with treatment, and practitioners feel more positive about the care they give. Stevenson (2002) makes the points that person-centred care does not necessitate a greater time element, that it has a positive influence on health outcomes, and that care can be more efficacious and compassionate as a result. He says that patient-centred care has been defined by six domains:

➤ the illness experience
➤ the context
➤ finding common ground
➤ partnership
➤ health promotion
➤ consultation limitations.

Vikas clearly wanted to find out about Swapna's experience of her illness and how it affected her life. However, he also needed to find some common ground, establish a partnership approach and carry out appropriate health promotion. He needed to do this without raising too high an expectation of what his service could provide, so that Swapna's own expectations were realistic.

Vikas would have felt that his use of time for this visit was well spent if he focused the care on Swapna's needs and what was important to her. The NHS Leadership Qualities Framework (2006) has often been used in the United Kingdom as a tool to develop leadership skills, for recruitment and selection and for career development. This focuses on three key areas, with five qualities for each:

➤ setting direction – seizing the future, intellectual flexibility, broad scanning, political astuteness and a drive for results
➤ delivering the service – leading change through people, holding to account, empowering others, effective and strategic influencing and collaborative working
➤ personal qualities – self-belief, self-awareness, self-management, drive for improvement and personal integrity.

This framework has been redeveloped as the NHS Leadership Framework (2011). It incorporates the same elements but delivering the service is seen as the central theme, with demonstration of personal services, setting direction, working with others and managing and improving services being the contributing elements. Creating the vision and delivering the strategy are seen as strategic elements that comprise part of the environment in which leadership exists and where leadership potential is maximised.

Vikas has a senior role in healthcare, and as such would be very aware of the importance of taking a lead in practice. He would be aware that health outcomes have to be measured and standards achieved, and that his time is finite with any patient. He would also recognise the need to set a direction or have a vision for his service, and be politically astute enough to be able to market his service to commissioners in ways that would meet the organisational goals of his employer. However, in terms of delivering the service that he was employed to do, he was aware of the need to be a change agent and to collaborate with others so that they felt empowered to influence care and strategies as much as possible. These qualities would have less immediate effect on his time with Swapna, but would ensure that he was able to be effective in his role of helping her take greater control of her health and her life. The qualities that Swapna would value most during Vikas's first visit would be his personal qualities: he needed to demonstrate to her that he had personal integrity and that he had the self-awareness and self-belief to improve her care. Once she was convinced of this, she could trust his professional expertise in relation to her health needs.

The resources that he needed in his role with Swapna were time and professional expertise to carry out health needs assessment and give appropriate advice, and his ability to collaborate with other services involved in her care to ensure that the needed changes in service provision actually took place.

Cornwell and Goodrich (2009) highlight the importance of focusing on patients' experiences of care in order to improve services. Nurses need to feel empowered to deliver care that they would want for themselves and their loved ones. This requires qualitative and quantitative measurement of what patients want, and every service needs to be aware of its importance. All nurses need to be involved in assessing whether patient needs are being met and what patients or clients actually want from their service. Swapna's needs will vary according to her health status, age and stage in her journey with cystic fibrosis, and these variations need to be taken into account and her care modified as appropriate.

The importance of measuring the quality of patient experience is also

discussed by Coulter *et al.* (2009), who warn that relying too much on quantitative measures and statistical indicators has the potential to disengage the
nurse from patients' feelings about their experiences. It would be possible for
Vikas to tick all the right boxes in terms of assessing Swapna's health needs and
give her appropriate advice, but still leave her unconnected with the process
and disempowered from taking an active part in her care. It could also leave
her feeling devalued as a person by focusing too heavily on her illness rather
than on her life and the opportunities to achieve her potential.

Gerry Bolger from the Department of Health, in his conference presenta-
tion (2009) on developing and understanding nursing indicators, highlighted
many quality indicators in relation to nursing care, as follows:

➤ accountability and responsibility
➤ ethical and legal integrity
➤ record keeping, reporting and monitoring
➤ equality and diversity
➤ leadership
➤ communication
➤ safety
➤ technical skills
➤ care and treatment
➤ education and training
➤ advocacy
➤ dignity
➤ humanity
➤ empowerment
➤ coordination, integration and continuity
➤ clinical reasoning
➤ patient involvement in care
➤ evidence-based practice
➤ person-centred care
➤ multidisciplinary and multiagency working
➤ contributing to an open and responsive culture.

Although not all of these nursing qualities might have been obvious to Swapna
during Vikas's visit, many would have been. His personal qualities of communicating sensitively, empowering her, being open and responsive to her needs,
recognising her diverse needs, involving her in decision making and demonstrating advocacy, dignity and humanity would have been clear, as would his

evidence-based technical expertise, clinical reasoning, focus on safety and his overall care and treatment. However, it might take longer for her to appreciate his ability to coordinate and work effectively with other agencies and take a lead in her care, educate others, keep accurate records, have ethical and legal integrity and be accountable for his nursing practice. Nevertheless, Swapna would undoubtedly feel confident that Vikas was an expert and compassionate nurse who valued her part in the care process, and would be able to help her feel confident in her ability to take greater control over her life and her health.

So far, we have discussed the relationship between resourcing and ensuring excellence in compassionate nursing and how this does not necessarily involve a greater time commitment. In the next section, we will go on to discuss how these resources are central to the care of people we nurse.

THOUGHTS FOR YOUR PRACTICE

- How do you ensure that the patient or client remains central to the care process when resources are limited?
- How do you know that your patients or clients are satisfied with the care that they receive and that their expectations are realistic?
- How do you bring about improvements to your service based on patient or client feedback?
- How do you think that you could enhance your contribution to setting direction for the service that you are involved in?
- How could you take a more active role in leading the delivery of the service?
- How do you use your own personal qualities as a leader of practice?
- How do you ensure that the previous three areas of the Leadership Qualities Framework are central to your leadership role?
- How do you assess whether you have the resources you need for a compassionate and caring service?

ONGOING PRACTICE – DISCUSSION ONE

Vikas knew how important it was going to be to build a trusting relationship with Swapna during this first visit. Swapna had challenging health issues to deal with, and yet she was very young. Most people her age did not have to worry about their health at all, and it must be difficult to enjoy activities which were normal for her age, or to socialise fully with others who had more choices about how to live their lives.

Vikas knew that the children's services were very supportive and were able to build strong relationships with children and young people and their families. It was not quite the same in adult care services, and Vikas constantly felt as if he was being asked to provide more than he was able to. His time was limited and so were the resources at his disposal. However, it was essential that Swapna felt he was someone she could trust, and someone who had the expertise to help maintain her independence as far as possible, with minimal need for hospital stays.

Vikas knew that many nurses felt stressed by having too many demands on their time and tended to distance themselves from patients as a result. However, in his experience those same people did not actually spend less time with their patients, and quite often needed to spend more time because patient anxiety levels would rise. He found that by *genuinely* caring about each patient as an individual, and keeping calm and appearing relaxed, often the patient would feel comfortable to discuss their issues more readily. Vikas felt that you could not fake caring about people; you either did, or did not, care about them as individuals. He knew that these were challenging times in terms of meeting the needs of people with shrinking resources. However, it was possible to balance patient need with achievable expectations and still achieve outcomes expected for his service. Vikas rang the doorbell and was genuinely looking forward to meeting Swapna.

How could the challenge of resourcing potentially have a negative impact on our relationship with patients and clients?

Vikas clearly was a caring and compassionate nurse, and he wanted to focus on his new relationship with Swapna. He knew that she was used to a high level of care from the children's services and that she would be feeling anxious about the change in service provision. He was the face of that service, and he needed to reassure her that her needs were important to that service too. He is clear that nurses should be genuinely caring, and that simply fulfilling the criteria for *appearing* to care was not enough for him in his nursing practice.

Compassion is not something that can be turned on and off at will, because that is not compassion at all. It is easy for practitioners to regard patients who expect to be treated with care and expertise as being demanding, as highlighted by Stearns (1991) in an American study. However, this can be more a reflection of how stretched and stressed practitioners are, rather than of expectations being too high. Every person has a right to nursing that is genuinely caring, and adopting a victim-blaming approach can be a way in which carers alleviate feelings of guilt for being unable to provide the care they would wish to. We suggest that it is a recipe for disaster for inadequate and uncompassionate care to become the norm in any environment and that it should be challenged at every level – by the patient, their loved ones, nursing colleagues, other health-care practitioners and managers, but most of all by nurses themselves.

A judgemental attitude towards patients in our care, or clients in our caseload, is wholly inappropriate. Wong (2004) says that 'The definition of a nurse, previously that of a healer and the bringer of relief where there has been suffering, has increasingly been superseded by the discourse of the cost-conscious nurse' (p. 7). Such a nurse thinks that they need to appear busy all the time, and talking to patients is not considered as 'being busy'. They also talk about 'nursing beds' rather than patients, and in some cases, 'bed blockers' when referring to patients who occupy beds for longer than is considered to be medically necessary. 'Emptying beds' can be seen as more important than the real nursing focus of getting someone to the point where they can safely go home. These are all derogatory ways of viewing patients and their care, and are resource-based approaches to patient care. Whilst Wong (2004) describes the care environment in Singapore, this managerialist approach has become the norm in many countries. Most patients do not want to be in hospital or feel that they are a burden on society or healthcare services. Swapna clearly did not want to be in this situation herself. Wong (2004) describes how nurses feel frustrated and compromised when their ethos of holistic care is at odds with the managerial pressure to deliver cost-effective care. Terminology such as 'demanding', 'decrepit', 'confused' or 'agitated' depersonalises the patient and is generally not an accurate indication of the patient's personality, but more of their behaviour in stressful circumstances, and as such cannot be justified.

Vikas had no such thoughts in mind when he met Swapna, though his role was very much to reduce the possibility of her needing to be rehospitalised because this is expensive for healthcare services and disruptive and distressing for the person involved.

We have discussed the relationship between resourcing and ensuring excellence in compassionate nursing and the potentially negative impact that resource constraints can have on our relationships with patients and clients. Now we will discuss how nurses can take a lead in influencing care so that compassion remains central, despite the challenge of resourcing.

THOUGHTS FOR YOUR PRACTICE

- Do you ever feel that patients or clients in your practice setting are labelled as 'demanding' when nurses are too busy to meet their needs? How do you think that you could start to change this mindset?
- How do you think you could minimise the effect that a cost-conscious environment can have on relationships with patients and clients?
- How can you have a positive impact on nurses labelling people and depersonalising their needs?
- How would you share these thoughts with others?

KEY THEME TWO – TAKING THE LEAD ON INFLUENCING RESOURCING

ONGOING PRACTICE – DISCUSSION TWO

Swapna was pleasantly surprised by Vikas's empathy throughout his visit. She had been used to a very caring service, but sometimes she felt that she was a small cog in the wheel. Her parents had always been worried about her, and their concerns tended to be the focus of many of the visits and appointments. Because she loved them very much and wanted them to stop worrying about her, she was glad that they had these opportunities to express their concerns. However, she was an adult now and she wanted to take more responsibility for own health.

Although she was still living at home and her mother answered the door to Vikas before she could get there, it was clear that it was Swapna he wanted to talk to. He said to her mother that he wanted to help Swapna to be less reliant on hospital-based care and that he needed to get to know her in order to understand her specific health needs. He said it would be easier if he talked to Swapna alone. He said it in such a caring way that she could tell that her mother did not feel excluded, but instead felt reassured by his caring approach towards her daughter.

It was also clear that he viewed her as an equal and was genuinely interested in her point of view and her concerns. It was a good feeling because she had never felt before that her views mattered. She was convinced by his questions and answers that he was very knowledgeable and skilled in the complex treatments and medications that she often needed. He also discussed ways that would help her to anticipate escalating health problems. He knew a lot of the people that she had been involved with. She gained confidence that he would be someone who could help her to stay as well as possible at home, and that she would be able to call on him if she started to feel more unwell.

What is our role in taking this lead?

Swapna's transition from child to adult services could potentially be very stressful, and Vikas was aware of that. The Confidence in Caring guidelines (DOH 2008, p. 28) lists the following qualities that patients want from healthcare providers:

➤ a care provider – who looks and behaves professionally: is caring, competent, knowledgeable and compassionate and provides holistic, timely, seamless care and information
➤ a care partner – who works with patients and relatives to plan care, gives constant feedback and reports, and helps them to navigate the health and social care system
➤ a champion – who puts their interests first and protects them when they are vulnerable
➤ a coordinator – who is constant, accessible and accountable for communicating the plan and monitoring the delivery of care.

Shapna was used to working with care providers and she was impressed with Vikas's caring and compassionate attitude, his holistic approach to her needs and his knowledge base. However, she was less used to being a partner in her care, and this was something that she wanted to embrace. She had never felt that she was the one who was navigating her way through the complexity of healthcare, as she was always directed by others. She felt that Vikas would champion her cause, and she was already very impressed with how skilfully and sensitively he had negotiated a one-to-one discussion with her, without her mother being present. He clearly knew people in the places that she went, and she felt that he would be a key coordinator of her care needs, if she was unable to coordinate her care herself. Therefore, in Vikas, she could see someone who would be just the nurse that she wanted in this new and alien adult healthcare environment.

From Vikas's point of view, he also felt that the visit had gone well. He felt that he had started to build a trusting and equal relationship with someone who was not used to being a partner in her own care. He was very aware of resource limits, but he felt that Shapna's expectations were realistic and that she wanted to avoid hospital admissions where possible. That in itself would save money in terms of expensive hospital care, which was an important measure of his success as a community matron. He knew that in this role, he used his skills and knowledge as a highly experienced nurse, and he used his heart, hands and head in his empathetic understanding of a patient's feelings and in the actual care that he coordinated. He also knew that he was a leader in practice, and that he needed to adapt his service to meet the emerging needs of patients who were living in their own homes with diagnoses and prognoses that were ever more serious and had severe acute deteriorations. As Bharj (2009) says, he had to think creatively to balance value for money and efficiency with a person-centred and high-quality approach. He had seen other nurses who were exhausted and stressed by this challenge, and they were unable to be clear advocates for their patients or leaders in improving the service that they led. He found that people did listen when he found reasons to adapt the service he gave, and he felt that he could be a powerful change agent for quality enhancement.

One approach to supporting nurses to become agents of change is the Productive Ward initiative in the UK (www.institute.nhs.uk). Although primarily focused on hospital-based care, this has tried to empower front-line staff to improve the quality of care in their environments by systematic processes that make the most of the time that they have and the resources that are at their disposal. Mumvuri and Pithouse (2010) discuss how this initiative was implemented in a mental health setting. 'Showcase wards' were identified through a competitive application process, and training and support was provided for nurses in leadership roles so that they could understand how they could make an impact on the organisational objectives. Clear outcome measurements of key target areas (identified by the ward teams) were audited and displayed as evidence of good practice. This had a positive effect, not only on patient care, but on staff morale, reduction of episodes of violence and aggression and on how valued and empowered staff felt. Other Productive Ward initiatives have enhanced leadership skills of staff and improved quality and efficiency. This has freed up time for more direct care and time to spend with patients, and has led to better teamworking, less stress and higher levels of morale and motivation (Ford 2010).

Leung (2008), in a Hong Kong study, says that interpersonal conflict can result in higher staff turnover and absenteeism, and conflict can also waste a great deal of time and make any service less efficient. This is particularly evident in times of complex and chaotic change. In these situations, leaders can underestimate the complexity of specific changes and focus on tools or processes, rather than on the effect on staff. Karp *et al.* (2009) say that at times like these, focusing on how staff relate to each other and react to change is crucial.

Arnold *et al.* (2008) discuss the problems of 'managing immature, irresponsible or irritating employees', and although we might not want to label colleagues in this way, we think that most people can identify with the problem of working with people who are less engaged than us. Improving staff motivation can be a real challenge; performance reviews and appraisals often do not help individuals to feel key to the change process or to achieve quality outcomes. Instead, they become individuals who have a negative impact on the morale of others. Because disengagement, demotivation and conflict at work can have such a strong detrimental effect on performance, a collaborative or cooperative approach is essential to achieving outcomes and providing high-quality care.

Helping people to feel motivated and happy at work can enhance the efficiency and quality of the service. If all members of the team feel actively engaged in achieving something that the organisation values, then they become more motivated towards success. If a man cleaning the building at NASA can feel that his main role is to help put a man on the moon, then every nurse should feel able to say that they are an important part in providing the best care possible, regardless of their grade or experience.

Some community-based services have piloted a Productive Community Services programme. It is clear that community nurses lose a great deal of time due to mismanaged referrals and poor discharge planning. Clover (2010) reports on a study of district nursing teams in London where each mismanaged referral was found to cost a district nurse an average of 5 hours of additional time – which no service can afford. Individual nurses can often identify the reason(s) for wastage of time and play a part in trying to bring about positive change. Duffin (2009) gives a clear example of district nurses doing this by examining their working practices and saving more than 5 hours a week. If the nurses involved are free to identify time-wasting components of their roles, then they feel part of the problem solving. This bottom-up approach is far more likely to bring about success than managerial victim-blaming calls to 'work smarter', which insult and demotivate hard-working nurses.

The Productive Ward and Productive Community Services programmes are based on the principles of lean thinking. Lean thinking is not about down-sizing or reducing services; it makes the assumption that doing things the hard way not only makes the service more costly but also tends to result in a poorer-quality service. The idea is that lean thinking will improve efficiency and quality without sacrificing either. In order to apply the approach, we need to understand what the main purpose of our service is and then assess our processes to find out if there are more efficient ways to deliver them. Womack and Jones (2003) say that lean thinking combines adapting to change with continual improvement and elimination of waste. We need to think about the least wasteful way to provide what our patients and clients want. A great deal of time and resources can be spent on things that the client or patient does not even know about, does not value and would not miss. Systems need to be evaluated by all members of the care process, including high-level manag-ers, healthcare assistants, domestic and cleaning staff and patients and carers themselves. We then need to think about what our circle of influence can be, and what change we could implement or influence.

Nursing is based on communication, something that can take a great deal of time or be just as effective in a briefer period. The Brief, Ordinary and Effective (Crawford *et al.* 2006) model of communication combines non-verbal communication such as eye contact, touching and smiling, with respectful and valuing comments, the appropriate use of questioning and cla-rifying, and confirming points. This can be carried out even in very complex situations, and in fact is even more important in these situations.

The Solution-Focused Brief Therapy (Berg 2003) approach focuses on solution building rather than problem solving. The focus is on how would you know that something has helped; what would need to change and what would things be like without that problem. Nurses who take either of these approaches can communicate more effectively in a shorter time, leaving the person involved feeling just as valued. These types of communication strat-egies can help save more time than those employed at present by some nurses when they are under pressure, which are based on avoidance of eye contact and 'seeming busy'. Patients and clients who have been at the receiving end of more negative communication often become more distressed and require more nursing time in the long run.

In other words, nurses can be more instrumental in making the best use of the resources at their disposal. If they feel that they have a major part to play in the organisational processes, as well as the patient care, they can bring about a great deal of positive change. As a result, they feel more valued and motivated, and patients and clients are happier with the service they receive. Vikas clearly felt like he was a leader of practice, as well as a care provider, and in what was actually a short time period, Shapna felt valued and supported by Vikas in a service with which she was unfamiliar.

Having discussed what our role could be in taking a lead in influencing resourcing, which is a key challenge in relation to compassionate nursing practice, we now go on to discuss exactly how this can take place.

THOUGHTS FOR YOUR PRACTICE

- Do you feel that you are able to fulfil your role as care provider, partner, champion and coordinator? If not, what could you do to develop these roles?
- How do you balance the need for cost-effectiveness with maintaining a high-quality, person-centred approach?
- How do stay as flexible and adaptable as possible to changing healthcare needs and expectations?
- How do you challenge inefficient and outdated practices?
- Could you think more positively in relation to reacting to change? How can you encourage others to do the same?
- How do you stay motivated in your role? What do you do to motivate others?
- Do you see yourself as a change agent? How could you bring about more change, particularly in relation to compassionate care?
- How could you develop your role in relation to becoming more involved in making processes more efficient?
- What is your own personal circle of influence? Is it greater than you think? How could you work on extending it?
- How could you be more effective in your communication when you have little time available?
- How could you take a more solution-focused rather than problem-centred approach? How could this help you to appear compassionate when time is limited?

ONGOING PRACTICE – DISCUSSION THREE

Vikas reflected on his time with Swapna as he was driving away. He knew that there was a growing number of young people who were surviving to adulthood with life-limiting conditions. Advances in medical care meant that life expectancy for people with conditions such as cystic fibrosis was greater than ever before, and there were many other medical conditions that necessitated young people transitioning from the children's to the adult services. These services were very different: resourcing for children tended to be greater, there was often additional money available from charities and ill children were much more appealing and emotive than older people with life-limiting or challenging health needs.

The movement of young people into the care of adult services could lead to expectations that were impossible to meet in the current financial climate. In addition, the process was not always as smooth as it could be. He knew that nurses from the children's teams tried to prepare young people for this transition 2 years prior to the change in service provision. They tried to build relationships and communication pathways with adult teams, but he knew that staff were often not very receptive to thinking about situations that were not part of their caseload as yet. Some of the patients might not survive to the point of needing care from adult services, which was sad, but this added to the problem of a potential lack of engagement from adult services.

Having met Shapna, Vikas felt that much could have been done to ease her transition; her anxiety would have been less and continuity of care would have been better. Greater teamworking across the services might even have prevented her recent hospital admissions. He knew that he needed to take a lead in trying to improve the experience of young people such as Shapna. This would also have a beneficial effect on health service resources, because unnecessary hospital admissions might be avoided. He decided that he would arrange to meet with the team leader from children's services as quickly as possible to try to agree joint processes and greater communication across the teams.

How can we take a lead in keeping compassionate care at the heart of nursing, despite resource constraints?

Vikas was clearly a compassionate practitioner who wanted to provide the best care possible for Shapna. However, he was also very clear in his mind about what his role actually was, and how the outcomes for his service were measured. As a community matron, he had a remit to reduce hospital admissions, which are the major users of healthcare resources. Therefore, he needed to get to know Shapna and assess her needs, so that he could advise her and provide her with strategies for maintaining her independence and care at home. This was also what Shapna wanted, because she disliked going into hospital and wanted to be as independent as possible and feel secure in her relationship with someone from the adult care services.

Although Vikas's role included a wider remit, his focus could still stay on Shapna, and his ability to be compassionate was not compromised by focusing on resource limitations. Every area of nursing practice is affected by resource constraints, and every nurse should be trying to provide outcome-measurable, cost-effective care. However, we do not think that this should be at the expense of poorer relationships with patients and clients. A great deal of nursing time can be taken up by administrative processes that are more time consuming than they need to be. Another poor use of nursing time is spent when teams are in conflict or there is ineffective leadership.

Stevens (2010) expresses real concern that nurses spend so much time collecting data to demonstrate the fact they are delivering high-quality care that they have little time to provide the care itself. As she says, we do have to be able to prove that we are providing high-quality care and meeting targets for healthcare; however, if systems are uncoordinated and inefficient, this wastes precious nursing time. Stevens (2010) says that she is bombarded with emails requesting data that will take her hours to provide, and that many nurses will identify with this pressure on their nursing time. She feels that this compromises the amount of time available to use her expertise and suggests that more organisations should use health economists, who are skilled at calculating whether processes and innovations improve productivity, as part of their clinical audit teams. Managers often do not have this expertise but are under pressure to provide statistics, and the data usually has to be provided in a hurry by busy nurses. This is clearly not a good use of nursing time; it might not give the information required to demonstrate quality care, and it clearly has an impact on time available for nursing care.

Time is one of our most valuable resources, but it is often not used to best effect when there are difficulties with team dynamics or conflict in the practice environment. Because conflict cannot be eliminated, leaders have to be skilled at managing it to minimise the impact on team dynamics, staff morale and motivation, and the time lost solving relationship-based issues and therefore not spent with patients or clients.

A study in Mississippi (Morrison 2008) highlighted the importance of emotional intelligence as a leadership strategy in managing conflict. Nursing is a highly stressful vocation, and occupational stress is a major concern, both for individuals and organisations, because it can lead to nurses taking time off sick, functioning below their level of expertise or leaving their posts. High staff turnover is very expensive in terms of recruitment and selection of new staff, and teams are left understaffed whenever a colleague leaves. Recruitment freezes are also common in times of financial hardship and unfilled vacancies can be seen as a management cost-saving exercise, and even when someone *is* appointed, the time taken for them to reach full work capacity has an effect on the workload of colleagues.

Therefore, keeping people well and happy at work, and having a motivating environment where everyone feels valued and valuable, is the most cost-effective strategy, organisationally, and the most beneficial for individuals working in that environment, and for the patients in their care. Morrison's study (2008) found that the emotional intelligence of leaders, in knowing how to minimise and deal with conflict, was key to improving interpersonal relationships in healthcare environments. The art of relationship management is essential when handling people's emotions in the highly charged and highly stressed environment of nursing. Leaders without these skills can inadvertently allow harassment, conflict and morale-reducing values and practice to become the norm, or may actively contribute to these situations.

Staff are the most valuable resource in healthcare, and the fostering of collaborative working and reduction of interpersonal conflict are key to the effective use of staff time. Farrell (2001), in his paper from Tasmania, refers to staff conflict as 'horizontal violence', which he says can happen on three levels. First, the micro-level in relation to one-to-one relationships between staff – many nurses have reported that intrastaff aggression is more traumatic than a patient assault (Farrell 1997, 1999). Second, the meso-level, which focuses on organisational structures and practices – although these are often in the control of nurses themselves, nurses can become disengaged, disenfranchised, disempowered and marginalised by negative organisational workplace practices. Third, the macro-level, which concerns interactions with other dominant groups, such as doctors. Conflict at any of these levels has an adverse effect on self-esteem. Roberts (1983) says that nurses, in common with other oppressed groups, can exhibit signs of self-hatred and a dislike of other nurses. Aggression can breed aggression, which can escalate problems and is likely to result in repetition of the aggressive behaviour, and an abrasive environment becomes the norm.

The focus on tasks-to-time ratio (Farrell 2001) means that nurses have to work at a certain speed and achieve a certain number of tasks within a given period in order to be accepted as part of the team. In addition, patients or clients can be reduced to the category of 'tasks', which can be reflected in terminology such as 'the appendix in Bed One' (Travelbee 1976). This has an effect on individual nurse autonomy, as well as having a negative impact on relationships with patients or clients.

Ensuring excellence in compassionate nursing care will almost inevitably not be possible in such a negative working environment where nurses feel that they need to conform and fit in for them to be accepted as part of the ward team. Furthermore, we believe that the care in such an environment is likely to be less cost-effective, as patients and nurses will be unhappy, and an unhappy environment is likely to have a negative impact on the health of all concerned.

Cornwell (2009) says that there are several reasons for needing the nurse's experience to be a positive one:

➤ It is the right thing to do, and healthcare organisations need to set the standard for being good employers.

➤ If staff are happy, the patient experience will be much more positive – 'where staff have good experiences, so too, it seems, do patients' (Cornwell 2009, p. 11).

➤ Poor standards in relation to quality and compassionate care can often be attributed to a lack of support from the organisation and individuals rather than 'bad staff' (Cornwell 2009).

➤ Staff retention and recruitment are likely to be enhanced where staff have good experiences. Organisations attract and retain a higher calibre of staff in these situations.

➤ There are real efficiency gains when there is a commitment to staff health and well-being, through lower sickness and absence rates, and reduced costs spent on recruitment and induction.

In addition, Cornwell (2009) highlights the importance of caring conversations, 360-degree feedback to give positive reinforcement and mentoring staff to show compassion towards themselves. Staff who are more critical of themselves, and less forgiving of their shortcomings, may become those who are unable to demonstrate compassion to others.

The importance of not exhorting staff to work harder or better is also seen as important by Cornwell (2009). As she says:

Most staff are likely to feel they are already working as hard as they can and to the best of their abilities. Asking staff to work harder may well have the unintended consequence of demoralising them and making it feel more difficult for them to do their daily jobs. Instead, leaders need to find ways to help staff to feel enabled to work competently and compassionately. In turn, this should improve their job satisfaction. (Cornwell 2009, p. 12)

Vikas undoubtedly felt valued both personally and professionally in his role. He was making a difference to patients on an individual basis, and to his organisation through meeting health outcomes. He was positive about his role and his part in the organisation, and felt a responsibility to be cost-effective and compassionate. Valuing himself, his patients and his colleagues was part of his personality and his work ethos, and this made him feel positive in his nursing role. He would, therefore, be a valued and cost-effective member of the organisation, and would be likely to stay in his role for some time. This would reduce the need for costly staff recruitment and education, which at his senior level would be considerable. So in his role, he was taking a lead in keeping compassionate care at the heart of his nursing practice, despite the strong focus on cost-effectiveness.

THOUGHTS FOR YOUR PRACTICE

- How do you balance focusing on the individual needs of patients or clients with the conflicting demands of your role?
- Are there ways in which you could reduce the impact of collecting work-related data so that you could use your nursing expertise to best effect?
- Have you experienced conflict in your practice environment? If so, why do you think this happened? How was it handled and by whom?
- How do you think that you could make your practice environment as motivating as possible, and do you think that this would reduce potential conflict?
- Think of examples of conflict at the micro-level, in relation to one-to-one relationships between staff. How could you reduce the potential for this level of conflict?
- Think of examples of conflict at the meso-level, in relation to organisational structures and processes. How could you reduce the potential for this level of conflict?
- Think of examples of conflict at the macro-level, in relation to interactions

with dominant groups of people you work with. How could you reduce the potential for this level of conflict?

- Do you sometimes feel as if you need to focus too much on tasks in order to get the work done, rather than on the patients or clients for whom you care? Is there anything more you could do to focus on their individual needs?
- Do you feel valued personally and professionally? How could you help other members of staff to feel more valued?

SUMMARY

We are in no doubt that resourcing is a major challenge to ensuring excellence in compassionate nursing care in the current healthcare environment. Staffing levels can be severely compromised, commissioners require value for money from the services they administer and nurses are required to demonstrate efficiency and cost-effectiveness in every element of their role. At the same time, a strong focus on quality of care and meeting the expectations of users of the service is also seen as paramount. The overwhelming focus on targets and outcomes can be detrimental to caring for people in the way that both nurses and people in their care would feel was ideal, and nurses feel criticised for being unable to provide the care they believe is optimal. This is the challenge for healthcare today. How can cost-effective, outcome-measurable care be combined with compassionate, caring and patient-centred care within the available resources?

In this chapter, we have used Vikas's approach to his role and Shapna's needs to illustrate how these issues can be central to care in a resource-constrained environment. We have explored the relationship between resourcing and providing compassionate care in several ways.

We have concentrated on the positive link between patient- or client-centred care and outcomes. The NHS Leadership Qualities Framework (2006) and the NHS Leadership Framework (2011) highlight the importance of effective leaders needing skills in relation to setting the direction of care as well as leading delivery of the service. The frameworks also highlight the importance of personal qualities of leaders in achieving a high-quality care environment. Leaders and managers in healthcare need to meet the challenge of reduced resources, while trying to reduce the impact of this on patients and clients. Quality indicators and quantitative and qualitative measurement are essential to this process because the patient experience is paramount to effective care. It is all too easy to blame patients for being too demanding when they are anxious, or when they voice their concerns about poor experiences of care. It is also easy to depersonalise the care that we give to protect ourselves from becoming too distressed by care that we know falls short of what we consider optimal. So how can we remain caring but also conscious of the costs of the service we provide?

Knowing what patients and clients value in any service is essential – they say that they want a care provider, care partner, champion and coordinator (DOH 2008). Commissioners want value for money and efficiency combined with person-centred, quality-driven care. The Productive Ward initiatives are designed to empower practitioners to review practice and make changes so that they have more time available for direct patient care, but we need to ensure that any time saved is used to do just this, not to carry out even more administrative tasks (Middleton 2010).

At all levels of nursing, as leaders we need to think about how we can use time, our most valuable resource, to best effect. Lean thinking focuses on continual improvement through adapting to change and eliminating wasteful use of time and resources. Continuing to do things the same way when circumstances change makes things harder for us as nurses, can be more costly and can result in a poorer care environment. Melanie Hornett (2010), executive nurse director at NHS Lothian in Scotland, says that 'Getting it right first time saves time and money.' This could apply to patient complaints and distress, and the effect of poor care on patient motivation and empowerment.

Crawford *et al.* (2006) highlights the importance of brief, ordinary and effective communication which combines non-verbal skills with respectful and valuing comments. This approach makes the most effective use of time and leaves the patient or client feeling most satisfied with the care that they have received. Solution-Focused Brief Therapy (Berg 2003) is another approach that maximises time spent with people and focuses on solution building rather than mere problem solving. Both these approaches can help nurses to deliver cost-effective care as quickly as possible while leaving patients feeling valued and unrushed.

As nurses, we need to concentrate on our circle of influence to decide to what extent we are capable of effecting change. We need to build our networks so that we can influence circumstances as far as possible, while still accepting that some things are not in our power to change. Bringing about effective change and enhancing the care of patients and clients is very motivating for us as nurses. We want to keep compassion at the heart of our care and our service, despite the resourcing challenges that we face, and need to take an active lead in balancing individual patient or client needs with a cost-effective service. We need to ensure that data collection does not have a negative impact on care, or at least minimise its impact as much as possible.

We also need to take the lead on reducing the potential for complex conflict situations. To do this, we need to be aware of ways in which conflict can arise in the workplace and become skilled in conflict management in relation to personal relationships, structural and organisational factors, and dominant people and groups with whom we work. It is essential that nurses, and others in our team, feel valued, both personally and professionally, so that a positive team environment can remain at the centre of our care. All employees deserve to be treated with respect, dignity and sensitivity, which are all elements of compassion (Chambers and Ryder 2009).

Taking the lead in ensuring that we develop this positive culture in our care environment is key to excellence in compassionate nursing care, and we will discuss this in our next chapter. 'We all have a leadership role in creating a practice culture where care that lacks compassion is not tolerated and where developmental opportunities exist to enhance compassionate care' (Chambers and Ryder 2009, p. 195).

REFERENCES

Arnold E, Pulich M, Wang H. Managing immature, irresponsible, or irritating employees. *Health Care Manag*. 2008; **27**(4): 350–6.

Berg IK. *Solution-focused therapy: an interview with Insoo Kim Berg*. 2003. Available at: http://psychotherapy.net/interview/Insoo_Kim_Berg (accessed 11 December 2011).

Bharj K. All staff should seize the opportunity to improve care. *Nurs Times*. 2009; **105**(42): 27.

Bolger G. Developing and understanding nursing indicators. *Second Annual Nursing Times Nursing Quality Conference Delivering High Quality Nursing Care*. 2009 Nov 18; London.

Bradshaw J. The concept of social need. *New Society*. 1972; **30**(3): 640–3.

Chambers C, Ryder E. *Compassion and Caring in Nursing*. Oxford: Radcliffe Publishing; 2009.

Clover B. District nurses stymied by system. *Nurs Times*. 2010; **106**(41): 2–3.

Cornwell J. See the person in the health professional: how looking after staff benefits patients. *Nurs Times*. 2009; **105**(48): 10–12.

Cornwell J, Goodrich J. Exploring how to measure patients' experience of care in hospital to improve services. *Nurs Times*. 2009; **105**(29): 12–15.

Coulter A, Fitzpatrick R, Cornwell J. *Measures of Patients' Experience in Hospital: purpose, methods and uses*. London: King's Fund; 2009.

Crawford P, Brown B, Bonham P. *Communication in Clinical Settings*. Cheltenham: Nelson Thornes; 2006.

Department of Health. *Confidence in Caring: a framework for best practice*. London: Department of Health; 2008.

Duffin C. Community nurses find an extra five hours. *Primary Health Care*. 2009; **19**(10): 8–9.

Farrell G. From tall poppies to squashed weeds: why don't nurses pull together more? *J Adv Nurs*. 2001; **35**(1): 26–33.

Farrell G. Aggression in clinical settings: nurses' views. *J Adv Nurs*. 1997; **25**(3): 501–8.

Farrell G. Aggression in clinical settings: nurses' views – a follow-up study. *J Adv Nurs*. 1999; **29**(3): 532–41.

Ford S. Productive Ward boosts leadership. *Nurs Times*. 2010; **106**(7): 2.

Hornett M. Opening speeches. *Inaugural International Conference on Compassionate Care*. 2010 Jun 9–11; Edinburgh.

Karp T, Thomas I, Tveteraas H. Reality revisited: leading people in chaotic change. *J Manag Dev*. 2009; **28**(2): 81–93.

Leung A. Interpersonal conflict and resolution strategies: an examination of Hong Kong employees. *Team Perform Manag*. 2008; **14**(3/4): 165–78.

Middleton J. Time to care must not be jeopardised by NHS job cuts. *Nurs Times*. 2010; **106**(45): 1.

Morrison J. The relationship between emotional intelligence competencies and preferred conflict-handling styles. *J Nurs Manag*. 2008; **16**(8): 974–83.

Mumvuri M, Pithouse A. Implementing and evaluating the Productive Ward initiative in a mental health trust. *Nurs Times*. 2010; **106**(41): 15–18.

Roberts S. Oppressed group behaviour: implications for nursing. *Adv Nurs Sci*. 1983; **5**(4): 21–30.

Sills E. Nurse intuition will be restricted if technology dominates care. *Nurs Times*. 2010; **106**(8): 13.

Stearns C. Physicians in restraints: HMO gatekeepers and their perceptions of demanding patients. *Qual Health Res*. 1991; **1**: 326–48.

Stevens J. If data collection were managed, nurses could focus on caregiving. *Nurs Times*. 2010; **106**(12): 9.

Stevenson A. Compassion and patient centred care. *Aust Fam Physician*. 2002; **31**(12): 1103–6.

Travelbee J. *Interpersonal Aspects of Nursing*. Philadelphia, PA: FA Davis; 1976.

Womack J. Jones D. *Lean Thinking: banish waste and create wealth in your corporation*. Kent: Mackays of Chatham; 2003.

Wong W. Caring holistically within new managerialism. *Nursing Inquiry*. 2004; **11**(1): 2–13.

www.nhsleadershipqualities.nhs.uk (2006) and revised www.nhsleadership.org.uk/framework.asp (2011).

www.institute.nhs.uk/quality_and_value/productivity_series/the_productive_series.html

CHAPTER 3

Creating a compassionate culture in practice – taking the lead

Overview of the chapter

Key theme one – creating a positive practice culture

- Case study 3.1
- How can the organisational culture influence practice?
- Thoughts for your practice
- Ongoing practice – discussion one
- What makes a positive practice environment?
- Thoughts for your practice

Key theme two – developing an emotionally intelligent culture

- Ongoing practice – discussion two
- What is the role of the team leader in creating an emotionally intelligent team culture?
- Thoughts for your practice
- Ongoing practice – discussion three
- What contributes to an emotionally intelligent team culture?
- Thoughts for your practice

Summary

References

OVERVIEW OF THE CHAPTER

In the last chapter, we discussed how resourcing issues can be perceived as a major challenge to caring for people in a compassionate manner. We suggested ways in which the impact of financial constraints can be minimised, and how time spent with people can have maximum impact.

In this chapter, we discuss another challenge that we see as hindering compassionate care – that of the organisational culture of the practice environment. In some practice areas, it can become the norm for patients and clients to be treated as mere depersonalised objects, and their care can be reduced to tasks to be accomplished. Judgemental attitudes can become normalised and a patient-blaming culture can develop.

In these environments, caring nurses feel disempowered to bring about change, and low morale, demotivation and high levels of stress and sickness can become the norm.

As we said in the introductory chapter, although newly qualified nurses clearly have ideals and intentions of delivering high-quality care, if they work in a practice environment where these ideals are not valued or practised by others, they become acculturated within a 2-year period, they become frustrated and experience burnout due to their ideals being unfulfilled. This can lead to nurses feeling disillusioned to such an extent that they change jobs frequently and may leave nursing altogether (Maben *et al.* 2007).

Therefore, the importance of the culture being a positive one cannot be overestimated, both for nurses and for the people in their care. According to Ross (2010), effective leadership at ward or unit level is the key factor in creating an environment where there is 'a culture of support within which organisational compassion can flourish' (p. 27). It is a crucial role of the team leader, and for everyone in the team, to take a lead in creating an environment where nurses feel nurtured and therefore feel able to demonstrate compassion to colleagues as well as patients or clients.

As the NHS Leadership Qualities Framework (2006) and the NHS Leadership Framework (2011) clearly identify, true leadership is about setting the direction for the service in order to deliver the service. For this to take place, the team leader has to have personal qualities which include the attributes of emotional intelligence and transformational leadership. Setting direction for the service involves having a level of political astuteness, seizing opportunities for developing the service and driving the service forward to achieve outcomes, while remaining flexible in order to meet the requirements of purchasers and users of the service. For this to happen, leaders need to focus on delivering the service by supporting others through change, empowering others and holding them to account, as well as working collaboratively and influencing strategies. The personal qualities of self-belief, self-awareness, self-management, personal integrity and a drive for improvement are key to succeeding in leading a quality-driven service.

In this chapter, we focus on how organisational culture influences practice and what makes a positive practice environment. We then discuss the importance of developing an emotionally intelligent culture in taking practice forward. The role of the team leader is paramount, but every member of the team has a part to play in this process. Transformational and emotionally intelligent leadership are crucial to developing a positive practice culture where staff and patients feel valued, and where only excellent and compassionate nursing care is the norm.

KEY THEME ONE – CREATING A POSITIVE PRACTICE CULTURE

CASE STUDY 3.1

Martin really did not see how he could carry on any longer trying to pretend that he was his usual cheerful and professional self. He had been working in the Medical Assessment Unit for the past two years and he really enjoyed his role. It was a challenge providing care to acutely ill patients in such a busy environment, with such a high turnover of patients. However, he felt that as a team they managed to provide genuine care to frightened patients and those who cared about them. This was accomplished, he felt, by strong relationships within the team, and a strong sense of purpose and commitment to high-quality care. He also felt that all members of the team provided real support to each other and to students who worked on the unit. He had a good relationship with Rumbi, the team leader, who was a key instigator of this positive team environment.

Martin had been struggling for some time with how he had been feeling. At times, he thought that he might be depressed and was trying to decide whether he ought to talk to his doctor about this. However, he knew that what was behind his self-doubt and feelings of hopelessness was his relationship with his wife. They had always been so close, but recently he had felt that she was distancing herself from him. This afternoon, when he woke up after a busy night shift the previous night, she finally told him that she had been having an affair. He was devastated by this, and did not see how they could remain together, but she had said that she still loved him and had stopped the affair because she wanted to be with him. He felt that his priority was to rebuild his relationship with his wife, instead of working the night shift tonight. He did not feel that he was safe to work anyway, because he felt so upset and his mind would be on the discussions he needed to have with his wife.

He decided to contact Rumbi to discuss what had been happening to him today and how he felt. With another team leader, he might have felt unable to talk about the true cause of his distress, and he knew that other nurses would have just said that they were unwell. However, he knew that Rumbi would be supportive and understand the importance of him taking time off to sort out his home circumstances as far as he could. Rumbi knew that he worked hard and was very motivated in his nursing role, and he had always felt valued and listened to. He picked up the phone.

How can the organisational culture influence practice?

Martin clearly felt very much part of the team on the Medical Assessment Unit and felt that he was working in an environment where he could be honest with his team leader, and that she would not judge him or feel that he was not committed to his professional role.

So what makes a working environment a place where individual team members feel positive and motivated, and what makes a successful team leader where the organisational culture is so positive? White (2008) says that workplaces are similar to the weather, in that they all have their own emotional temperatures. This emotional temperature, or climate, can involve high energy levels, with high levels of motivation, where people want to work hard and develop. Alternatively, a work environment can make people feel stressed, angry and undervalued, and willing to do only the minimum. The result can be a constant state of irritation, impatience and irritability, which is not conducive to teamwork. We said in the previous chapter that conflict in the workplace wastes valuable resources in terms of time, but an underlying negative emotional culture or climate can also mean that people work well below their level of competence and capacity. White (2008) says that emotions are contagious and that it is important for a team leader to set the emotional climate by being positive, as this creates a positive energy. A team leader who is anxious, tense or miserable will cause others to behave in this way, and the whole emotional climate of the practice environment will affect both the staff who work there and the patients or clients in their care. This negative mirroring of mood was highlighted in relation to patient care in our previous book:

> As nurses, we need to be aware that if we seem tired, bored, uninterested, tense or in a rush then this will have a negative effect on the relationship with patients. In addition patients could start to mirror the mood that they think they see in their healthcare practitioner, which cannot fail to affect the amount of information that they are prepared to divulge and the way that they view the interaction and nursing care overall. (Chambers and Ryder 2009, p. 32)

If a negative emotional climate pervades the workplace, the potential adverse effect on patient care is clear. However, if a team leader is positive, encouraging and valuing, the whole mood of the workplace will be enhanced greatly. Positive environments can also cause mirroring of others' behaviour and positivity is contagious. Not all team leaders set the highest emotional temperature, and this can make an anxious leader even more anxious and tense. White's (2008) insightful paper describes how a descending spiral can develop whereby the more tense a manager is, the more anxious and debilitated staff become, which results in poorer performance and less productivity, which in turn makes the manager even more anxious. As we have said throughout this book, we all have a part to play in leadership, and it is possible that as individuals we could have a positive impact on the practice temperature and climate. White (2008) discusses how we could maybe smile more, use more positive body language and try to avoid looking anxious, all of which will help to enhance how we feel, and hopefully how others feel too when they are in our presence. We can also protect ourselves a little better from others' negativity by making a conscious effort not to mirror their facial expressions and body language.

Organisational culture has been likened to the personality of an organisation:

> Culture is comprised of the assumptions, values, norms and tangible signs (artifacts) of organization members and their behaviors. Members of an organization soon come to sense the particular culture of an organization. Culture is one of those terms that is difficult to express distinctly, but everyone knows it when they sense it. (McNamara 2000)

It is possible for a nurse to act very differently in one practice environment than in another, because the organisational culture might influence their beliefs and values – if they feel valued, their levels of motivation are likely to be much higher. The importance of inspirational leadership cannot be overestimated, for all members of the team to achieve their potential, for organisational goals to be met and patient care to be at the highest standard. Hemmelgarn *et al.* (2006) clearly link organisational culture and climate with the quality and outcomes of patient services. This paper says that staff who are more highly committed and experience higher levels of job satisfaction are more likely to provide a high-quality service, whereas staff who do not feel this way are more likely to make inappropriate decisions, fail to act as a team, experience emotional exhaustion, and the associated high staff turnover and poor work attitude will have a strong negative influence on quality of care.

An example from Australia of a positive organisational culture is Mater Health Services, where the emphasis on 'exceptional people, exceptional care' is clearly demonstrated through their organisational values:

➤ mercy – the spirit of responding to one another
➤ dignity – the spirit of humanity, respecting the worth of each person
➤ care – the spirit of compassion
➤ commitment – the spirit of integrity
➤ quality – the spirit of professionalism (www.mater.org.au).

Mater Health Services clearly markets itself on the core values above and gives every indication that it is striving to be a compassionate organisation, with a compassionate culture and climate towards both staff and patients.

The work of Dewar *et al.* (2010) on emotional touchpoints, which we discussed in Chapter 1, is an example of how a compassionate organisational culture can be further developed in relation to patient feedback. When nurses were approached with the patient perspective, using the emotional touchpoint of the situation and the emotions that they had felt as a result, they were much more likely to view these as interesting points for practice development, rather than as criticisms of the service or them individually. In addition, a tool was developed (Dewar and Ogilvie 2010) to capture individual staff perspectives on what was important to them in their working environment. Questions were asked about what made them feel positive within their work, what helped them when they were feeling a bit low, what sort of environment they liked to work in and what made them feel proud or valued. Knowing how individual staff feel, what motivates them and responding to those feelings is an important part of creating a positive organisational climate. Staff feel more supported and are more supportive to others, and they give and receive more praise. Staff working in a compassionate culture would therefore, in our opinion, be much more likely to be compassionate towards patients or clients in their care. The whole emphasis is then on creating a culture where all nurses take an active role, and a lead, in creating this environment.

Nolan *et al.*'s (2006) Senses Framework identifies six senses in relation to caring relationships, which we discussed in Chapter 1. These are clearly essential to patients and clients feeling valued, but are also key to nurses feeling valued. Nurses feel a sense of security and feel free of criticism and secure in their conditions of employment. In addition they feel that their employer recognises that the emotional demands of their roles are stressful, and they feel that they work within a supportive but challenging culture. Their sense of continuity is maintained through clear communication about expectations and standards of care. They have a sense of belonging because they feel part of a team with a recognised and valued contribution to make, and a clear sense of purpose with therapeutic vision and goals. Therefore they feel a sense of achievement in their ability to use their skills to their maximum, so they also feel a sense of significance in that their role and their part in the whole care process is valued and important.

Martin clearly felt all these things, and the organisational culture of the unit was a positive one. Rumbi played a key part in creating that positive emotional climate.

Tomey (2009) discusses how some organisations and workplaces can be unhealthy places to work. They can have high levels of sickness, work-related accidents, stress, disputes and complaints and low levels of work performance, productivity and motivation. Tomey (2009) says that in the workplace, 'Poor leadership and management styles; impatient, defensive, unsupportive leadership; lack of supervision and guidance; control; and a lack of recognition of contributions have been identified as major stressors' (p. 16).

Wong and Cummings (2007) reinforce this point and say that developing transformational leadership in nursing is an 'important organizational strategy to improve patient outcomes' (p. 508).

Transformational leadership strategies and staff-focused environments empower others. These involve such leadership traits as positivity and accessibility together with listening skills and collaborative working strategies which help build trust. Transformational leadership involves visionary and charismatic leaders who excite and energise their teams. It also puts a strong emphasis on valuing people, encouraging the same vision and pride, building trust and inspiring others to perform beyond their expectations. In comparison, transactional leadership merely focuses on tasks and getting the tasks carried out. Tomey's (2009) paper clearly links transformational and participative leadership with healthy and happy workplace environments and healthy patients and happy staff.

Alimo-Metcalfe and Alban-Metcalfe (2006) discuss transformational leadership as having three main dimensions:

➤ leading and developing others – which involves showing general concern, enabling, being accessible and encouraging change
➤ personal qualities – which include being honest and consistent, acting with integrity, being decisive, inspiring others and resolving complex problems
➤ leading the organisation – which involves networking and achieving, focusing on team effort, building shared vision, supporting a developmental culture and facilitating change sensitively
 (pp. 299–300).

In our case study, Rumbi probably demonstrated all these skills at different times. Martin felt that he could discuss his personal issues with her in relation to his work role, an indication that she took an active role in leading and developing others by showing genuine concern and being accessible. She also had personal qualities which made her appear approachable to Martin, and she had a clear idea of the importance of sensitivity in helping members of staff to feel important and valued members of the team. Rumbi also exemplified a 'nearby leader' rather than a 'distant leader' (Alimo-Metcalfe and Alban-Metcalfe 2006) because she was charismatic and had positive characteristics, such as 'being dynamic, sociable, open and considerate, original and sensitive' (p. 296). They identified a high correlation between the leadership style of the leader and the culture of the organisation or the practice area and concluded that 'the most important responsibility of leadership, is to create the most appropriate culture for the organisation' (p. 307). However, they also emphasised the fact that leadership cannot remain the sole responsibility of senior managers and that all members of staff at all levels and in all parts of the organisation must take a lead in taking the service forward.

With such emphasis on the relationship between leadership and the practice culture, who are the good leaders and managers in today's healthcare environment? Often, nurses who do not hold a management role feel that they do not have a part to play in being innovative and developing new ideas.

Is this because they are not being encouraged to think in this way?

Kennedy (2008) found in a Welsh survey that there was a lack of ability in many organisations to identify and nurture future nurse leaders. She makes the point that in industry, senior managers are expected to identify future leaders, and that their own career progression depends on this. However, this is not common in healthcare environments. In fact, developmental opportunities for nurses often lead to frustration and demotivation for those who have taken part in these initiatives. When they try to take their ideas back to their practice areas, they often find that their passion and enthusiasm for change is thwarted, and that managers feel threatened by the challenge of new ideas, not energised to take a lead in developing them. This attitude needs to change in order for new ideas to be generated, and for them to take root and genuinely enhance care.

Kennedy (2008) discusses a Welsh initiative launched in 2008, called Free to Lead: Free to Care, where the focus was on empowering ward sisters and charge nurses, because they were perceived as key change agents, yet the support for them to develop their ideas and their leadership skills was variable. This initiative recognised the key role of the nurse manager in relation to the experiences and outcomes of a patient's hospital stay, and on the standards of care being delivered within their practice area. Kennedy (2008) says that there can be a lack of communication between healthcare personnel or between these staff and patients, which can sometimes result in a lack of compassion. Nurse leaders and managers have to be able to identify and solve problems and have effective strategies to reduce the level of chaos and cope with the complexity of care.

The allocation and effective use of resources is key to success in coping with this complexity and in ensuring that patients receive the care that they need and deserve. Kennedy (2008) cites an old proverb which says 'It's tough trying to keep your feet on the ground, your head above the clouds, your nose to the grindstone, your shoulder to the wheel, your finger on the pulse, your eye on the ball and your ear to the ground.' However, she says that this ability to be a contortionist is key to high-quality leadership and care. Managers are often recruited into leadership positions because they are excellent practitioners, and yet they receive little help in making this vital transition into their new leadership role.

According to Martin (2007), great leaders are able to think in an integrated way so that they can identify solutions to complex problems. They do not see the problem in isolation but look for what factors are relevant in causing the problem, so that they can see the relationships between these factors and causes and develop innovative solutions. The importance of thinking in this way is key to effective leadership.

One simple way of getting to the root of a problem quickly is by reflecting on challenging situations by using the '5 Whys' (www.mindtools.com), a technique developed for the Toyota Production System in the 1970s. It tries to get to the root of the real problem by asking 'why' with respect to the presenting problem and working backwards until the eventual cause of the problem comes to light. It might not work in very complex situations, and might lead to false assumptions, but it is quick and easy to use and is surprisingly effective in many situations.

Using a public health nursing example:

➤ Why is Tina desperate to be rehoused? Because she says that her house is too crowded for her, her partner and their three children.
➤ Why is she feeling that the house is too crowded when she has three bedrooms? Because the youngest child, Jack, is sleeping in the same room as her and her partner Jason.
➤ Why is it a problem that Jack is sleeping in their room? Because he cries at night when Jason comes in from a night out.
➤ Why does he cry at night only when Jason has been out? Because Jason drinks too much when he goes out with his friends and he is noisy when he comes in.
➤ Why does this worry and affect Tina so much when it only happens a few nights a month? Because Jason is physically abusive to Tina on these nights and he has threatened to harm Jack if he carries on crying.

Therefore, the real problem is not the size of the house but the fact that Tina is worried for Jack's safety when Jason has been drinking, and that the domestic abuse in their relationship is escalating. Even if it were possible to move into a larger home, this would not solve the domestic abuse or allow Tina to feel that she and her children are safe in their own home. The public health nurse needs to be able to discuss the domestic abuse with Tina, rather than concentrate on the presenting problem that Tina always raises, which is the size of the house.

From the acute nursing perspective, another example could be:

➤ Why is Patience crying? Because she is in pain following her knee replacement 2 days ago.
➤ Why is she in pain when she has regular analgesia prescribed? Because she is an hour overdue for her medication.

➤ Why is she an hour overdue for her medication? Because the drug round is late.

➤ Why is the drug round late? Because there has been nobody to dispense drugs for the past hour due to a staff handover which has taken up much of this time.

➤ Why does a staff handover mean that a medication round is delayed? Because the only people able to dispense drugs are involved in the handover.

In this situation, the fact that all of the nurses able to dispense medication are involved in the handover is identified as the real problem in relation to Patience's distress. Persistently asking 'why' can determine whether all nurses involved in the handover actually need to be, and further, what other strategies could be used to ensure that medications (and presumably other important areas of care) are not neglected because of the nursing agenda taking priority over patient care.

However, it is important to acknowledge that using this approach with patients or clients, or in fact with students or teams, can feel quite challenging. We suggest that it can be best used by individual practitioners, or team leaders, to help identify the true source of a problem as the first step to finding a solution. Alternatively, it can be used for team discussions, or student action learning circles, as long as the 'why' questions are asked from within the group, rather than by outside facilitators, mentors or team leaders. The emphasis needs to be on genuinely searching for possible causes of a problem from a questioning perspective, rather than a challenging approach – which could lead to defensiveness and distress.

Rumbi did not need to use this approach with Martin, because he felt open to discussing his particular personal problems. However, if Rumbi was trying to identify why a particular team member was struggling with a part of their work remit, she might find the 5 Whys a helpful technique. However, she would need to use the approach carefully, on her own and alongside other strategies, because she might be completely wrong in her perceptions of potential causes for behaviour or skills deficits.

As already stated, transformational leadership is key to inspired nurse leadership. Covey (2006) discusses how management is about 'doing things right', whereas leadership is about 'doing the right things', and Govier and Nash (2009) say that the 'care of people' should be central to effective leadership. This involves treating people with respect, demonstrating high standards of nursing practice and being a caring role model for others, whether they be patients, clients or members of staff. This basic humanity needs to be demonstrated in *all* workplaces, but especially those where staff are involved with stressful and emotional situations, such as those that nurses encounter every day. Govier and Nash (2009) discuss the challenge for executive nurses in 'taking the bedside to the boardroom' (p. 25); in other words, balancing the business and financial needs in a caring and sensitive environment. Inspiring and influencing others is key to enhanced productivity and performance of staff, and to outcome-measurable services that are identified as high quality by both staff and patients. This is particularly important in the complex dynamic and business-focused environment of healthcare today.

Effective role models are essential in nurse leadership and in delivering compassionate care. How can student nurses and more junior members of a practice team understand the importance of compassionate care if they do not see this exemplified by their more senior colleagues? Firth-Cozens and Cornwell (2009) say that affiliative behaviours, such as holding a patient's hand, or showing caring facial expressions, are important aspects of role-modelling compassionate care towards patients. Similarly, effective role-modelling can be demonstrated through compassionate and supportive behaviour towards colleagues. This encourages others to demonstrate compassion in their practice and reduces the potential for burnout, 'compassion fatigue' and stress. In our case study, Rumbi was clearly being an excellent role model, and therefore was able to create a compassionate environment in which to work.

Ethical leadership is key to the leadership process, and Northouse (2009, pp. 157–70) identifies six elements of ethical leadership:

➤ the character of the leader – trustworthiness, respect, responsibility, fairness, caring and citizenship
➤ the actions of the leader – showing respect, serving others and showing justice
➤ the goals of the leader – appropriate and ethically sound goals
➤ the honesty of the leader – presenting the reality of the situation while being aware of how it could affect others
➤ the power of the leader – appropriate and positive use of power and influence
➤ the values of the leader – kindness, altruism, responsibility and accountability, justice and a sense of community.

These elements are a real challenge for any nurse leader to maintain in today's challenging environment. However, they are important skills and character-istics for anyone with a genuine interest in taking the nursing service forward in a compassionate and dynamic manner. Being a leader carries with it a great deal of responsibility in terms of ethical decision making. The health and well-being of vulnerable people is in the hands of nurses. Strong, effective and compassionate leadership is key to ensuring a safe, caring and outcome-measurable service within available resources.

Inspiring and motivating nurse leadership involves many different char-acteristics in potential leaders. Palfrey *et al.* (2006) stress the importance of leaders and managers being ethical. They cite the importance of Gillon's (1994) ethical attributes relevant to medical practice, which are 'honesty, equity, impartiality, respect and a high level of competence' (Gillon 1994, cited in Palfrey *et al.* 2006, p. 65). They also stress the importance of value-based principles listed by the Nolan Committee (1995) of 'selflessness, integrity, objectivity, accountability, openness, honesty and leadership' (Nolan 1995, cited in Palfrey *et al.* 2006, p. 65).

Westwood (2010) uses the 'nine Cs' of inspired nurse leadership as her framework for leadership. These are communication and negotiation, clarity, consistency, connection, coaching, compassion, courage and confidence, cre-ativity and cheer (or complimenting yourself and others).

Wedderburn Tate (1999) stresses that leaders need to welcome challenge, encourage a work–life balance, be resilient, be prepared to accept that they cannot always be successful, be politically astute and have a highly attuned sense of when to trust and act on advice and information, and be emotion-ally stable. She says they may not necessarily be the most intelligent person in the organisation and might not see themselves as a leader, but they do stick to their priorities while still responding to changing circumstances. However, their personal attributes of being well attuned to people and being able to give and receive positive feedback are often particularly key to their success-ful leadership.

Whichever theoretical perspective you find helpful (*see* Table 3.1), all these characteristics contribute to creating a positive and compassionate practice cul-ture through inspirational leadership.

TABLE 3.1 Characteristics of ethical and inspirational leadership

Northouse 2009	Gillon 1995, in Palfrey 2006	Nolan Committee 1995, in Palfrey 2006	Westwood 2010	Wedderburn Tate 1999
Character of the leader		Selflessness Integrity	Courage and confidence	Welcome challenge Resilient Intuitive about when to trust people and information Do not always know that they are leaders
Actions of the leader			Communication and negotiation Coaching Creativity Cheer (or compliments)	Encourage work–life balance Concentrate on objectives Give and receive compliments
Goals of the leader	High levels of competence	Leadership	Consistency Clarity Connection	Political astuteness
Honesty of the leader	Respect Honesty	Openness Honesty		Emotional stability, and IQ. IQ is not necessarily the most important attribute
Power of the leader				Accept they cannot always win
Values of the leader	Equity Impartiality	Objectivity Accountability	Compassion	

It is useful to re-evaluate ourselves against key leadership attributes on an ongoing basis to ensure that we have not become complacent and that we are reaching our own potential as leaders. We need to be aware of changing circumstances, changing relationships and changing priorities on our ability to demonstrate inspired leadership.

It is important to create and sustain a vision and to communicate this to others in order to motivate them to work towards this vision. One of the clearest examples of inspirational visions is that of Martin Luther King (cited in Northouse 2009, pp. 92–3) in his famous 1963 'I have a dream' speech. Visions are based on clear values and a clear pathway of what needs to change in order to achieve that vision. Inspirational nurse leaders need to be able to articulate what excellent and compassionate practice is, and ensure that they create a culture where such a vision can be at the forefront of practice.

THOUGHTS FOR YOUR PRACTICE

- What do you feel is the emotional climate of your practice area, and how important is the role of the team leader in creating and maintaining this climate?
- How do you think that you could play a greater part in developing an even more positive climate in your practice area?
- How do you think that your patients and clients feel about the organisational culture of your workplace? Could this be affecting the quality of their experience and patient outcomes?
- Can you identify the key organisational values in your practice area? Could you influence these at all, if you feel that a shift in values would be beneficial?
- How is feedback – from patients, clients and staff – incorporated into development of the service? Is this feedback valued, and does change take place as a result? If not, how can you help develop this process?
- How can you see the Senses Framework helping to make staff feel valued in their practice roles?
- How do you think that you could develop even greater transformational leadership qualities?
- How do you think that new leaders could be identified and supported within your practice area?
- Think of a problem that exists in your practice area and use the 5 Whys to try to determine possible root causes. Does this approach help you to address this problem?
- Can you become an even more inspirational role model to colleagues and students? If so, how?
- Do you feel that leadership is always ethical in your practice area? If not, what do you think would help you to enhance practice-based, ethical leadership?
- What inspirational leadership characteristics can you see in leaders in your practice area? How can you further develop these characteristics yourself?

ONGOING PRACTICE – DISCUSSION ONE

Rumbi was not really surprised to hear from Martin, as she had been worried about him for some time. Although he was still the same professional and sensitive practitioner that he had always been, it was clear that he was far from happy in his life generally.

Rumbi believed strongly in working collaboratively as a team; if one member of the team was unhappy, then it potentially affected the whole team and the care they provided. In any case, how could nurses who spent their working lives caring for others not be concerned when a colleague was struggling? She knew that many nurses in management roles would concentrate on staffing their wards, rather than face the individual situations that affected their staff. However, that was not how she worked, and she felt that her colleagues' approaches contributed to unhappy and stressful working environments. She remembered that when she was newly qualified and working in a ward where everyone seemed too busy to show an interest in their colleagues' lives, the nursing care had been some of the worst that she had ever experienced. Staff sickness and turnover was high, and the ward sister seemed to be instrumental in increasing the stress and decreasing the morale of those who worked there. She resolved at that time that she would try always to be interested in her staff and how they wanted to develop in their professional roles.

In her discussion with Martin, he was very honest about his personal circumstances and she expressed genuine regret for how he was feeling. Rumbi told him to concentrate on his home situation and said she would make sure that his shift was covered. She could sense his relief at her response and knew that he would return to work as soon as he was able to, and that he would continue to be a valuable and hard-working member of the team.

What makes a positive practice environment?

We have discussed the importance of organisational culture on influencing practice, and in particular how essential inspired leadership is in this context. We will now focus on what makes a practice environment a positive place for both patients and staff.

Braynion (2004) discusses how managers and leaders are instrumental in setting and maintaining the norms, acceptable behaviours and ways of interacting within an organisation – in this case, the Medical Assessment Unit. Martin clearly felt comfortable divulging deeply personal issues to members of his team, and to Rumbi, perhaps because this was typical of the ongoing behaviour and type of communication within the team. Rumbi was clearly playing her own part in leading a team where this was considered to be the norm. St Pierre and Holmes (2008) highlight how power and disciplinary strategies that are designed to control, disempower and oppress staff have a strong negative impact on motivation and morale.

McGregor (2006) discusses two different theories in relation to staff motivation. First, Theory X, in which employees are perceived as disliking work, having no ambition or responsibility and generally unintelligent or at least gullible: they would rather follow than lead, resist change and are self-centred and unconcerned about organisational goals. If Rumbi had considered Martin's situation from this perspective, she would have seen him as being selfish in not coming to work, as trying to avoid work and as having no concern for patients in his care. She would then have tried to persuade him to come in and cooperate with her goal of getting him to work his shift. She might have tried to emotionally blackmail him into coming to work by saying how his patients would be disadvantaged. She might even have resorted to threats such as putting negative comments on his staff file. This could have had the desired but short-term effect of Martin working his shift – though possibly with errors occurring because of his emotional distress. The same approach with other staff would probably have meant that they worked as little as possible that shift, and generated increased hostility, disengagement and low morale.

McGregor's Theory Y assumes that staff consider work to be as natural as play and rest, and that people are self-directed as long as they are committed to organisational goals. People are assumed to be creative, ingenious and able to handle and actively seek responsibility. In this scenario, Martin would be assumed to have personal goals that matched organisational goals because he would want to feel self-fulfilled at work. As Rumbi had already treated him in this way, he would feel fully committed to returning to work as soon as possible, and would take time off only if this was absolutely necessary.

Lees (2009) differentiates between the mentality and motivation of nurses who merely turn up for work and those who focus on doing the job really well and contribute actively to effective teamworking. Motivation to deliver high standards of care needs to be nurtured in nurses who have been in nursing for some years, or who intend to make nursing a long-term career. High-quality care is dependent on motivated and engaged nurses, so it is important for nurse leaders to foster this motivation in their teams.

McClelland and Burnham (1995) say that the most motivating managers have emotional maturity, little egotism and a democratic, coaching style of management. In addition, Burnham (1997) says that 'achievement-motivated individuals, as McClelland's research has repeatedly demonstrated, do not require a meaningful sense of purpose to be energized to act. They require goals that are challenging, yet achievable through an individual's efforts and under his/her own control' (p. 8).

Martin clearly was self-directed and motivated at work, and to treat him otherwise would have been demeaning, unfair and potentially demotivating. Interestingly, McClelland (1962) also suggests that this achievement motivation approach works not only with individuals and organisations, but also with countries and the world as a whole.

McClelland and Burnham (1995) say that individuals have a need for achievement, power and affiliation. Martin clearly derived satisfaction from his achievements at work, had adequate power and felt sufficiently affiliated to the team and trusting of them to divulge his personal difficulties.

For nurses, keeping motivated and retaining a sense of job satisfaction can be a real challenge in today's target-driven and high-pressure environment. What makes people feel satisfied with their role, and their job overall, is highly variable from person to person.

For one nurse, it could mean that throughout their working day they know what they are doing, with minimal intervention from others. For that nurse, predictability during their working day is important, along with finishing their shift on time and having shifts that allow them to plan their domestic arrangements with certainty. Another nurse might want greater variety and challenge, and ability to influence their working environment. They might want to have professional development opportunities that enable them to move into higher-level roles as quickly as possible. Others might want to learn more about leadership, or might enjoy mentorship and want a recognised teaching aspect in their role.

Such diversity can pose a challenge for nurse leaders. A mix of healthcare personnel of different genders, ages, ethnicities, cultures and levels of expertise brings diversity to a team that is very positive for team dynamics and patient experience, but can also be a source of misunderstandings if some individuals do not feel that they are being valued and respected as much as others in the team. For example, nurses of different ages are likely to have different value systems, and these can create tensions in the workplace which affect recruitment and retention of staff. Swearingen and Liberman (2004) say that 'In the past, members of different generations were aligned based on seniority and years of experience. The oldest members of the workplace directed the youngest' (p. 55). However, this has changed, and older nurses are not necessarily the most experienced or the most senior members of the team. Swearingen and Liberman (2004) differentiate between the workplace expectations of veterans (born 1922–43), baby boomers (born 1943–60) and Generation Xers (born 1960–80). Most Generation Xers would not consider that unpaid overtime was a reasonable expectation from any employer, and they would expect to be consulted concerning managerial decisions. On the other hand, baby boomers and veterans might have different expectations and be more respectful of position or years of experience of others. This can lead to intergenerational conflict, and along with different motivational systems can be a challenge for a team leader. Farag *et al.* (2009) suggest that nurse managers need to reflect on how to interact with individuals from different generations, and also ensure that there is generational representation in the development of policies to maximise a flexible and inclusive work environment. In a Belgian study, De Cooman *et al.* (2008) conclude that if we intend to maximise recruitment and retention, generational and gender differences need to be taken into account. If financial constraints and organisational restructuring are not handled carefully, interpersonal connections and altruistic ideologies can be sacrificed, which could be detrimental to the care provided. As they say, 'For example, under strict budget constraints, increasing wages at the expense of time providing care and comfort measures for patients does not seem to be a good idea in view of the work motivation' (De Cooman *et al.* 2008, p. 63). This is an interesting point, because clearly in this study, which focuses on newly qualified nurses, standards of nursing care and being able to carry out nursing care well were valued higher than financial incentives.

Going back to our case study, it was important that Rumbi took on board the differing needs of nurses within her team. What was important to a male nurse with family responsibilities might be very different to a nurse of a different generation from either gender. In addition, personal characteristics and value systems might vary considerably from person to person within the team.

Therefore, it is really important for team leaders and managers to know what motivates different members of their team in order to try to increase job satisfaction as much as possible for everyone.

Job satisfaction has a direct effect on whether staff stay in their role, and on levels of staff turnover (Park and Kim 2009, Pillay 2009). It is essential, on a personal and organisational level, because happy staff are more engaged and tend to outperform less happy members of staff. In addition, organisations with high staff turnover do not use their resources to best effect because recruitment is expensive in terms of time and money. A destabilised team with high staff turnover due to low morale will be even less satisfied with their working environment, which will reduce productivity of existing staff. New members of staff need time to evolve into their new roles. This can result in the team being depleted, less productive and overstretched, from the time someone declares their intention to leave until their successor is fully functional and able to engage in positive team dynamics.

So for a team leader, it is essential to try to create a stable team where staff can have specific roles and feel valued for their area of expertise, and where positive team dynamics enable people to feel happy and supported. This is particularly important at times of great organisational change, when levels of dissatisfaction, burnout and absenteeism can increase, causing individuals to feel less empowered, which can also increase staff turnover (Kuokkanen *et al.* 2007).

Ritter (2011), in an American study, highlights the dangers of an unhealthy workplace environment. She clearly links a healthy and happy work environment with retention of nurses and positive patient outcomes in acute settings.

A positive organisational culture is created, developed and maintained by individual team members, but more specifically by the team leader. AbuAlRub and Al-Zaru (2008) clearly state the importance of recognising both performance and achievement with respect to staff retention and minimising job stress. Individuals who do not fit in can become stigmatised, in which case they lose reputation and credibility and are often denied developmental opportunities (Paetzold *et al.* 2008). The team leader is key to creating a workplace environment where nurses want to be employed and where they want to continue working (Ritter 2011). Therefore, the culture of the environment is crucial to recruitment and retention of staff.

In our case study, Martin needed to feel valued in his professional role and have stressors, such as his present domestic situation, to be acknowledged. Rumbi was clearly a supportive team leader who was able to provide him with this feedback and support. This would make him feel even more positive about continuing to work in this team in the future.

Commitment to care is another important factor in a positive practice environment. Cornwell (2010) says that a patient's experience of care is full of seemingly small incidents which might make them feel devalued, disempow-ered or uncared for. A nurse needs to actively engage with what constitutes good care for *specific* patients in order to identify ways of enhancing care for *all* patients. A nurse leader needs to clearly prioritise patient care in order for indi-vidual nurses to feel that this is part of the culture of the practice environment. More than this, nurses need to feel that it is unacceptable for anything other than high standards of nursing care to exist. If there is a persistent problem that regularly affects patient experience, nurses need to feel empowered and motivated to think about possible solutions. Nurses also need to feel 'cared about'. Remote and uninterested managers who do not listen to their staff have often been found in areas where poor care has been reported (Cornwell 2010). This again highlights how essential it is that leaders have high levels of self-awareness as well as advanced communication skills to enable them to engage effectively with others. Therefore, the links between caring about staff, on the one hand, and good patient or client care, on the other, are clearly crucial. As Masterson and Gough (2010) say, leadership occurs within a rela-tionship, and as such it is a relational act. They say that 'It is the way leaders transform relationships that, ultimately, transform services' (Masterson and Gough 2010, p. 23).

The complexity of nursing leadership is demonstrated through Cook's model (1999, cited in Cook 2001), where he says that this involves four elements:

➤ experience – what the nurse leader brings to their role
➤ understanding – what the leader understands about what they do
➤ external environment – organisational structures and culture prevalence
➤ internal environment – what beliefs and values are held by the leader.

Cook says that clinical nurse leadership is focused on 'continuous improve-ment through influencing others' (2001, p. 46), and this is based on ability to implement change, formulate evidence-based solutions, exercise clinical judge-ment and be professionally autonomous and accountable. This is a formidable challenge for any leader – any nurse wanting to be a credible and effective leader needs to be assertive in moving their service forward in relation to organisational goals and through collaborative working. They need to be able to empower others to take on leadership roles in their teams. They need to be able to use different relational skills, in different circumstances, with a diverse range of people who are internal and external to their teams. They need to be supportive of more junior members of the team and students who are based in their practice areas, giving people as many developmental opportunities as possible so that they too can develop as leaders. They need to be effective role models and focus on developing evidence-based and patient-centred care, where nursing care is competent and safe. However, more than this, they need to develop a practice culture where patients, clients and nurses in the team feel cared for and cared about. Leadership should not be about hierarchical position but about the personal qualities of the leader. Confidence, empathy and consistency are key to being a leader in practice.

Nicholls (1994) writes about the 'heart, head and hands' of transformational leadership, where the 'head' is concerned with creating a vision and a positive culture within an organisation; the 'hands' is about supervisory competence and the ability to be flexible in different situations; and the third component, the 'heart', is about engaging with others and inspiring them. Through the use of the 'heart', strategic and supervisory leadership becomes inspirational and transformational and is therefore raised to a higher level.

In our case study, we know little about Martin's practice environment, but what we do know is that Martin does feel motivated and empowered to carry out his nursing in a caring and compassionate manner. He also feels supported by Rumbi and is able to discuss his distressing personal circumstances with her. So it would appear that Rumbi is a transformational leader who is leading with her head, hands and heart.

Having discussed the importance of creating a positive practice culture and how this benefits nurses, patients and clients, we now want to focus on the role of emotional intelligence in creating a positive culture within any given practice environment. An emotionally competent and emotionally intelligent team can work together to maximise the use of resources and enhance the nurse and patient experience within the care environment.

THOUGHTS FOR YOUR PRACTICE

- In your practice area, how does your team leader influence the culture of your working environment? Does this influence have a positive or negative impact overall? Could you influence this culture to a greater extent yourself?
- Can you think of examples of when managers have used Theory X and Y motivational styles? How did these styles impact on your level of motivation?
- Think of ways in which you could develop greater Theory Y approaches in your leadership role.
- Have you worked in practice environments in which you have felt

greater motivation? How did this affect your performance, your level of empowerment and feeling part of the team? Think of ways in which you could enhance your motivation of others in your practice environment.

- What motivates you in your professional role? Do you feel that your team leader appreciates the differences between what motivates you and what motivates others in your team? How can you use this knowledge in your own leadership role?
- Can you think of ways in which being valued for your specific expertise and role has made you feel more motivated at work? Can you think of times when this approach has helped maintain team stability? How could you develop this approach to a greater extent?
- Think of ways in which you could increase feedback on how people carry out their roles and not just on what they achieve.
- Is there sufficient recognition of personal stress and individual circumstances in your team? How could you help develop a culture where the personal needs of individual team members are taken into account to a greater extent?
- Do you think that your team leader is sufficiently focused on the nature and quality of care in your practice environment? How could this emphasis be further enhanced? How could you take a greater role in developing this increased emphasis yourself?
- Do you have an inspirational leader? Do you think that you are an inspiration to others? How could you inspire others to an even greater extent?

KEY THEME TWO – DEVELOPING AN EMOTIONALLY INTELLIGENT CULTURE

ONGOING PRACTICE – DISCUSSION TWO

Rumbi thought about the conversation with Martin once they had finished talking. Martin was an excellent nurse who was very committed to high standards in nursing care, and he was also very supportive of other members of the team. She knew that he would have made the same decision if he was in her position, and that other members of the team would be very concerned about Martin's situation, once they heard.

As a team leader, Rumbi considered that providing good patient care was the responsibility of individual team members. However, as a nurse herself, she knew how important it was for people to feel valued in the work environment. She believed that nurses who feel appreciated, valued and are happy undoubtedly are more compassionate and caring to patients, and health outcomes are consequently better. An important part of *her* role, therefore, was to create a supportive environment where each nurse felt valued, appreciated and supported. She recognised that life is not always predictable, that traumatic situations and serious illness are unfortunately part of life and at times personal situations seriously impact on people's ability to work in the way that they normally would. It was her responsibility to ensure that despite these events, care was safe and of a high quality. Ensuring that nurses were supported and listened to enabled her to assess when stress levels created pressure points that were unsafe. She was also aware of when *she* was particularly stressed and she had colleagues that she could talk to at such times. So her priority was to create an environment where nurses and patients felt as relaxed and as calm as possible. She hoped that Martin could solve the problems that he had at home and looked forward to him returning to work.

What is the role of the team leader in creating an emotionally intelligent team culture?

We discussed the importance of emotional intelligence in relation to compassionate nursing care in our first book, *Compassion and Caring in Nursing*, and stressed it again in Chapter 1 of this book, particularly in relation to nurses having a passion for their role in order to be effective leaders. The potential influence of emotionally intelligent team leadership on a practice environment culture will be discussed in this section, and again in Chapter 4 when we discuss a leader's positive attributes.

Positive relationships in teams are key to effective working. The way to achieve them according to Cummings *et al.* (2008) in their Canadian study, is through relational leadership. They say that 'Relational leadership, leadership that influences outcomes for providers and patients through building and maintaining relationships in the nursing workplace, is founded on a theory of emotionally intelligent leadership' (p. 509). They state that their research has shown that this style of relational leadership is associated with lower levels of fatigue and exhaustion in nurses and higher levels of job satisfaction, emotional well-being and relationships with other nurses and healthcare professionals. In addition, nurses seem to be able to meet patient care needs more effectively when they work in a relational leadership environment. The links between relational leadership, excellent nursing care and a positive working environment were evident through:

➤ visible nursing leadership – nurses felt more supported to be innovative.

➤ nurse managers consulting with staff – nurses had greater opportunities for staff development and felt that they had greater support in managing conflict.

➤ good working relationships between physicians and nurses – nurses had greater staff development opportunities, were able to participate in strategic decisions, felt more autonomous and felt that they had sufficient resources to provide quality care.

➤ a clear philosophy of nursing – nurses felt more able to take part in policy decisions and felt more able to be innovative (Cummings, *et al.* 2008, p. 514).

This study by Cummings *et al.* (2008) clearly identifies that the culture of the environment can have a strong influence on positive working relationships and can increase staff satisfaction and reduce burnout. Some factors are able to be adapted and changed: leadership style, staff development opportunities, resourcing appropriate nursing positions and encouraging autonomy and decision making can make a real difference to staff satisfaction and patient care. Cummings *et al.*, in their previous study (2005), say that 'emotionally intelligent leaders inspire by engaging emotions, passions and motivations that reveal the possibility of achieving goals that might not otherwise be seen. They work through emotion to mobilise teams, coach performance, inspire motivation or create a vision for the future' (p. 3). In our case study, Rumbi is clearly able to understand the emotions, stresses and stressors of others in her team and is therefore able to help develop a more positive work environment where people feel valued and understood. Goleman, who has written the seminal texts on emotional intelligence, says that emotions spread very fast and that:

> When people feel good, they work at their best. Feeling good lubricates mental efficiency, making people better at understanding information and using decision rules in complex judgements, as well as more flexible in their thinking. Upbeat moods, research verifies, make people view others – or events – in a more positive light. That in turn helps people feel more optimistic about their ability to achieve a goal, enhances creativity and decision-making skills, and predisposes people to be helpful. (Goleman *et al.* 2002, p. 17)

So the links are clear between emotional intelligence and leadership, where emotions need to be understood, and job satisfaction and high performance valued. Groves *et al.* (2008) have carried out research into whether it is possible to deliberately develop emotional intelligence; working with business studies students in California, they proved that this was possible across the full spectrum of emotional intelligence. This provides strong evidence for the value of training programmes to help individuals and teams develop these skills. Another study carried out by Stubbs Koman and Wolff (2008) found that a team leader's level of emotional intelligence greatly influenced group-level emotional intelligence, which related strongly to team performance. Increasing opportunities for nursing staff development in relation to emotional intelligence might be a worthwhile use of resources, because it is likely to be an effective means of enhancing team performance and therefore of patient or client care.

Lucas *et al.* (2008) also support emotionally intelligent leadership in relation to nurse empowerment and the delivery of high-quality care. However, they say that if managers have too wide a span of control, then their ability to influence nurses in this way is significantly diminished. So it would seem to be important for managers to have a sufficiently small sphere of influence and for nurses to be enabled to become as emotionally intelligent as possible on an individual and a team level to mediate against this.

Akerjordet and Severinsson (2008), in a Norwegian study, found that a positive work climate – characterised by resilience, innovation and change – was created by empowered nurses led by emotionally intelligent leaders who were self-aware and had high supervisory skills. Freedman (2007) reinforces this and says that an emotionally intelligent leader increases customer satisfaction – in our case patient satisfaction and quality of care – through a process that involves:

1 an emotionally intelligent leader
2 creating an environment with higher-quality staff who make better decisions and who employ self-management skills
3 these members of staff feel more useful in their team
4 they consequently work harder and better
5 therefore, customers are more positive (Freedman 2007, p. 66).

Freedman (2007) also says that it is important to manage our emotions on three levels: at an individual level (within ourselves), on a relational level (with those we meet regularly) and on an organisational level (within the larger organisational structure). This creates a positive climate, which in the case of nursing influences patient care, retention of staff and staff performance. Six factors that influence the climate of a work environment, according to Freedman, are:

➤ leadership – level of commitment to their leaders
➤ alignment – level of organisational engagement and sense of belonging
➤ adaptability – level of ability to change
➤ collaboration – level of communication and problem solving
➤ accountability – level of motivation, responsibility and follow-through on commitments
➤ trust – level of faith in the organisation and their leader (Freedman 2007, pp. 215–16).

Without trust, it is questionable whether any of the other factors would have a positive effect or whether a positive climate would even be possible. In our case study, Martin clearly trusted Rumbi, was motivated to work to a high standard and could communicate with her and other team members. In addition, he was committed to Rumbi as a leader, and to the organisation in which he worked, and would probably have been flexible to meet the needs of patients and organisational goals. Rumbi herself also tried to be an effective leader who aspired to create a sense of belonging, flexibility, problem solving and motivation where members of her team could trust her and the organisation. This is the essence of emotionally intelligent team leadership, where practice can be as high a quality as possible, and where it is flexible and can change as the organisational environment changes.

In the next section, we will discuss the factors that contribute to an emotionally intelligent team culture.

THOUGHTS FOR YOUR PRACTICE

● Can you see elements of relational leadership in your practice environment? Can you think of possible ways in which these could be strengthened?
● Think of ways in which relational leadership could have an impact on the excellence of nursing care and the general working environment in your practice area.
● Is there clearly visible nursing leadership in your practice area? Do you think this could be strengthened, and could you take a role in this?

- How could nursing staff be consulted to a greater extent about strategic decisions? Could you increase your participation in decision making?
- Are the working relationships in your practice area positive ones? Could these relationships be enhanced in any way? If so, how?
- Do you feel that there are sufficient staff development opportunities for you and your colleagues? Can you think of any developmental opportunities that are not available? If so, do you feel able to suggest these to your team leader or manager?
- Do you feel that you work in a climate of resilience, innovation, change and empowerment? Can you suggest ways to further develop this climate?
- Think of ways in which you interact on an emotional level as an individual, in your relationships with others and on an organisational level. Can you identify ways in which these interactions could be even more positive?

ONGOING PRACTICE – DISCUSSION THREE

Martin returned to the unit that morning; in the end, he was away for only one shift, and had a couple of planned days off after that. He had spent the time with his wife and they tried to work out what had been missing from their relationship. They knew that they both still loved each other; she had started to have the affair because she was missing what she had valued in their relationship in the past. They made worthwhile plans to improve their relationship and Martin felt like a weight had been lifted off his shoulders.

When he came back on to the unit, he felt able to tell others about his situation, and other members of the team were very supportive. In addition, Rumbi had taken the time to ask him how he was and had been very pleased to see him looking so positive. He felt invigorated and even more positive about working in such a supportive team where a real team spirit existed. He knew that each member of the team felt supported and valued, and therefore was committed to providing excellent care to patients. He strongly believed that if members of a team were able to discuss their problems together and support each other, they in turn could be more effective role models in giving empathetic care to their patients.

What contributes to an emotionally intelligent team culture?

Martin was clearly working in an emotionally intelligent team where valuing of others was a priority. As we discussed in Chapter 1, Goleman *et al.* (2002)

say that emotional intelligence incorporates personal competence, in the form of self-awareness and self-management, and social competence in the form of social awareness and relationship management. We also said that the culture of a workplace or organisation is influenced by those who work there, but is predominantly set by those in strong leadership positions, and Sparrow and Knight (2006) reinforce this point. They suggest that 'Where there is a sense of apathy within an organisation, staff morale will be very low and customer satisfaction poor' (p. 184). This link between apathy, morale and patient satisfaction is key and it can be difficult to ascertain where the cause and effect factors lie. Does the apathy cause low morale and patient satisfaction, or vice versa? In some ways, this does not really matter, because all these factors are symptoms of a negative cultural environment.

Emotionally intelligent leadership is a skill that can be learnt once an individual recognises its importance and actively works towards developing it. Rumbi might not have always had such strong leadership skills, and she would not have suddenly acquired them when she moved into a team-leading position. It is far more likely that she was an emotionally intelligent leader even when she was working within the team. It is important that nurses develop these skills early in their careers and in their practice roles, because it is then more likely that they will be perceived as a leader and be able to make a positive difference in their work environment, as well as be in a better position to accelerate their career progression.

The team ethos, according to Sparrow and Knight (2006), is affected by:
➤ the level of emotional intelligence in individual members of the team
➤ the emotional intelligence level of the team leader
➤ the emotional intelligence level of the wider organisation
➤ historical factors that have affected a team or individual's emotional intelligence.

They also say that an emotionally intelligent team exudes attitudes and behaviours which demonstrate:
➤ motivation and commitment – to the team and the shared goals
➤ conflict handling – respectful challenge which encourages innovation
➤ team climate – positive feedback and appreciation of each member of the team
➤ self-management – empathetic awareness of others' needs in the team
➤ relationship management – healthy relationships and support
➤ openness of communication – sharing of thoughts and feelings

➤ tolerance of differences – diversity of experience and personality is seen as an asset and a focus of shared learning (p. 224).

Martin was clearly committed and motivated towards the team and what it was trying to achieve. He felt valued and able to communicate his own personal difficulties in the knowledge that he would be supported by both Rumbi and the team.

However, working as a team can be problematic. Teams are usually made up of very different individuals, who can have different values, expectations and objectives, and relate to others in complex ways. This complexity is compounded by the complexity of the healthcare environment, which often involves interprofessional and interagency teams, all of whom have different cultures and priorities and all of whom are vying for the limited resources available. This can mean that people stay in their professional silos and do not work collaboratively with others. However, as Robbins and Finley (2000) say, teams save money, increase productivity, improve communication and can achieve more than other working groups can alone. The better use of resources, in addition to higher-level decision making and higher-quality care, can create a wider vision and better strategies. 'Teams differentiate while they integrate', according to Robbins and Finley (2000), through blending people with diverse skills, which again means that resource needs can be lower. There can be professional barriers to teamworking, where different goals, professional mistrust, competition for status and power and a misunderstanding of roles can combine to create a tinderbox of tension. The organisational structures and systems can also conspire to make networking and communication very difficult. This can result in a culture of blame, where creativity and innovation are stifled, organisational goals are mismatched, stereotypical beliefs persist and an abdication of responsibility is the norm. This creates a 'toxic team', where there is too much competition, and a team tyranny can develop which forces individuals to do things the same way. In addition, mob behaviour can combine people into undesirable 'teams' with mismatched goals, where conflict is much more likely.

In such an organisational culture where conflict thrives, an individual's ability to think rationally is impaired and communication becomes ineffective. People who usually function to a high level become unable to do so because they are preoccupied with small issues; they become resistant to change because they are unable to see other perspectives. In a situation where conflict persists, it is even more important to use emotional intelligence to manage your own emotions and stay calm. You need to manage your own attitudes and behaviours in order to effectively manage the situation. It is essential that leaders can separate the people from the issue and define the actual problem in order to generate possible solutions, negotiate options and eventually solve the problem and resolve the conflict.

A team leader first has to decide whether to intervene or not; sometimes simply monitoring the situation can be more effective than taking action because the problem is temporary or resolves on its own. Hill's model for team leadership (Hill, in Northouse 2007) differentiates between whether the problem relates to tasks that need to be accomplished or whether it is the result of relational issues. Once this has been established, it is important to discern whether the issue is an internal or external one. If the issue is internal and task orientated, the most effective way forward is to focus on goals, structures that bring about the most positive results, good quality decision making, training and monitoring of standards. However, if the problem is still an internal one but more relationship orientated, then coaching, collaborating, managing conflict, building commitment, satisfying needs and modelling principles would be more effective. If the problem is external and environmental, identifying external stressors and finding ways to support and buffer people from them would be appropriate. Whichever approach is most applicable, problems need to be addressed and team leadership needs to be effective in order to obtain the best outcome. Even if there is no need for the team leader to intervene, informed team members can usually resolve the issue. If there does need to be intervention, maybe questions need to asked: is the issue task or relationship orientated, is the task clear, are expectations clearly expressed, are processes and strategies in place to enable positive decision making and are the team members sufficiently skilled, engaged, committed and satisfied? Regardless of whether the issue is internal or external, is it limited to the team, and are there clear networks and systems to support the team in the organisation?

Robbins and Finley (2000) list various problems that impact on team intelligence:

➤ mismatched needs
➤ confused goals and cluttered objectives
➤ unresolved roles
➤ bad decision making
➤ uncertain boundaries
➤ bad policies and stupid procedures
➤ personality conflicts

➤ bad leadership
➤ bleary vision
➤ anti-team culture
➤ insufficient feedback and information
➤ ill-conceived reward systems
➤ lack of team trust
➤ unwillingness to change (pp. 23–4).

Team leaders need to address these potential issues in their workplaces to ensure that there is a positive team culture and that team learning is possible.

A learning organisation is one where people want to work and where the morale and the quality of care is high. Senge (1990) suggests that learning organisations, are 'organisations where people continually expand their capacity to create the results they truly desire, where new and expansive patterns of thinking are nurtured, where collective aspiration is set free, and where people are continually learning to see the whole together' (p. 3). Nurses want to create nurturing environments where patients and clients thrive and feel both cared for and cared about, where patients feel safe and where their chances for recovery and health are maximised through evidence-based practice. Creating a learning organisation is paramount to achieving these goals and aspirations. If a team learns together, far more can be achieved.

Smith (2001) says that 'In situations of rapid change only [organisations] that are flexible, adaptive and productive will excel' (p. 2). He makes the point that individuals' capacity to learn is not in question, but that their work environment can negatively affect their opportunities to reflect on practice and feel engaged with quality improvement. Having a strong mental model of what high-quality care would consist of within a practice area, building a shared vision of that model and then jointly working out how to ensure that it happens is essential to team-learning success. Senge (1990) suggests that this involves leaders being able to articulate a vision and values, and to take responsibility for leading that vision forward by helping others to understand its importance.

When resources are severely constrained, a great deal is required of leaders who are, rightly, tied up with the day-to-day reality of providing a care environment which is safe and therapeutic. Pilgrim and Sheaff (2006) say that an additional constraint is that people who are influential in terms of policy and decision making rarely want to publicise the problems within their organisation, so it becomes difficult to truly learn and move practice forward. As they say, 'The current working solution . . . is that NHS organisations are permitted, nay encouraged to learn, but not too much and not too openly' (Pilgrim and Sheaff 2006).

When low standards of care hit the headlines, it is very distressing for all concerned. Nobody who works for an organisation wants negative publicity reported in the media, and most nurses are distressed by situations that lead to this bad publicity. The Francis Inquiry's (Francis 2010) damning report into the severe shortfalls in care at Mid Staffordshire NHS Foundation Trust in the UK raised extreme concerns about nursing leadership, and various hospital trusts have stated that these leadership issues are still a concern a year later. Leadership training is one of the casualties of reduced finances (Santry 2011), and ward managers are finding that they are unable to free up time to spend on their management roles. Therefore, there is a real risk of other tragedies occurring similar to the Mid Staffordshire situation due to failures in implementing the findings of the Francis Inquiry (Francis 2010). The NHS ombudsman, Ann Abraham, says in her report (Abraham 2011) that a change of culture is needed across the NHS to address the unnecessary pain, indignity and distress that older people are suffering, where even fundamental aspects of care are not being met. Her findings revealed an 'attitude, both personal and institutional, that fails to recognise the humanity and individuality of the people concerned and to respond to them with sensitivity, compassion and professionalism' (p. 7).

Learning from past mistakes or lack of care is a feature of a learning organisation. However, inadequate resourcing to support leadership roles that could focus on these problems, and a lack of educational opportunities to develop or enhance leadership expertise, frustrate organisations' attempts to be considered centres of learning. This, in turn, means that poor care and mistakes are even more inevitable. There are examples of nurses trying to address this problem by using different strategies to enhance care. One approach is by collecting positive feedback from patients – examples of quality care or improvements to care – to increase staff motivation and help them see their part in the quality improvement process (Ashton 2011). Empowering nurses to take a role in enhancing care and patient satisfaction is essential to high-quality care. Wang and Ahmed (2003) also see that organisational learning is crucial, but suggest that while individual learning is a significant factor, other factors are also important. These involve:

➤ individual learning
➤ right processes and systems

➤ a learning culture
➤ management of knowledge
➤ continuous improvement (Wang and Ahmed 2003, p. 10).

Nash and Govier (2009) state that team reflection, where support and challenge co-exist, has a positive impact on team effectiveness and on staff well-being and stress levels. Although using time for team reflection does take time away from actual clinical care, this is essential in today's fast-paced but low-morale healthcare environment, if positive change is to occur. As they say, 'Evidence and research show that taking time to [reflect as a team] . . . improves team effectiveness. Since this has a direct correlation with team member well-being and quality of care, the question is not can we afford to do it but rather can we afford not to do it?' (Nash and Govier 2009, p. 24).

An example of team learning is the Schwartz Center round. This is a multi-professional forum where those who are involved in giving care can discuss the difficult social and emotional issues that arise in caring for patients. Although it was developed in Boston, Massachusetts, the concept is now being piloted in two hospitals in the UK and in over 100 other healthcare environments, including nursing homes, health centres and outpatient departments across America. The round involves a monthly 1-hour session that provides an opportunity for healthcare professionals to reflect on their experiences and gain support and insight from others. Kenneth B Schwartz founded the Schwartz Center after being diagnosed with terminal cancer. He wanted to strengthen the potential for 'human connection', which was so important to him throughout his illness. His moving story clearly identifies his need for humaneness from the people he was interacting with following his devastating diagnosis (Schwartz 1995). Cornwell and Goodrich (2010) discuss how the King's Fund Point-of-Care programme supports the implementation of these rounds in the UK. They say that 'There is mounting evidence to support the assertion (DOH 2009) that staff who feel their organisations are supportive working environments, and their health and well-being are considered important, are able to deliver high-quality compassionate care' (p. 11).

Nursing is highly emotionally demanding, and this is often not addressed in the fast-paced and resource-driven healthcare environments of today. For example, it is not unusual for nurses to have no opportunity for debriefing and reflecting, even after the traumatic loss of a child in their care; they may well have had to deal with difficult, complex clinical care before the child's death, while simultaneously focusing on the physical and emotional needs of the child as well as that of the parents and others who loved the child, who are now experiencing terrible grief and loss. Whether death has been anticipated for a while, or is the consequence of unexpected clinical problems, in all such situations nurses will be called on to give of their utmost. Likewise, the death of an adult could be traumatic, unexpected or particularly distressing, or involve the loss of someone the nurse had grown particularly close to. The nurse could have experienced a recent personal loss which triggered extreme emotions. In situations like these, it is commonly expected that a nurse will simply carry on with the next nursing task that needs to be done. Do we make sure that students, who are essentially in our care, have a chance to address the emotional side of their personal experience of death? Do we do the same for our colleagues, and does anyone allow *us* to have an opportunity to express our grief? If this does not happen, we suggest that emotional burnout, extreme stress and low morale are inevitable, with resulting negative impact on our ability to deliver compassionate care.

There are many other demanding and upsetting situations, too diverse to capture here – feelings of depression or maybe even suicide, extreme anxiety, inability to bond with children or family, victimisation by an abuser – when a nurse has to dig deep to find inner reserves to carry on their role. We all know which situations are most difficult for us, as individuals, to cope with. Are your colleagues aware of these? Does your manager know? The first awareness of the seriousness of what we are feeling may be when we cannot face getting up in the morning to go to work, or when we start to cry in a way that surprises us, or when we become unaccountably angry with someone. As for noticing the stress in others, it may not be until they go off sick, or announce that they are leaving their post or the entire nursing profession. Does the emotional load of our caring role have to get to this point, or can something be done to help ourselves, and each other, before this? Do we notice when someone is becoming increasingly distressed, or is emotionally shutting down? What strategies are in place to help in these situations?

It is possible to miss early signs of emotional distress in ourselves and others, in our need to 'get the job done', but as leaders in practice we need to take responsibility for ensuring that our own emotional needs are met, as well as those of our colleagues within the work environment. In our case study, Rumbi was aware that Martin was reaching the point where his home situation was causing him too much stress to be able to work effectively. She knew that he needed to deal with his domestic worries in order to be able to carry on being the excellent nurse that he was. Nurses are notoriously bad at caring for themselves, and each other; someone going off sick increases the load on everyone else, so it is tempting to treat another's inability to come to work in a very negative way; for example, by trying to encourage them to come in anyway, by demonstrating a lack of understanding, by being critical or by using draconian measures to account for sickness and to discipline those who are sick. There is no doubt that some people *are* work-shy and not committed to their roles, teams or patients, and such situations do need addressing for the sake of other staff and patients in their care, but we do not always have the best performance management strategies to deal with them.

As leaders, we need to ensure that caring strategies are in place to help those who care for others. The Schwartz round approach is one way to allow people to take time out of their busy working lives to reflect on difficult and emotional situations in their day-to-day lives. The fact that it is a multiprofessional and multiagency forum that involves people at all levels in the organisation is a particular strength. Another strength is the diversity of people who attend, such as chaplains, administrators, allied health professional, nurses, doctors and healthcare assistants. The Goodman Research Group (2008) says that in America, people who have attended Schwartz rounds have said that their ability to provide compassionate care has improved, as has multiprofessional teamworking. In addition, policy changes have been made which have enhanced care. They say that they feel better supported, less isolated and less stressed as a result of attending these rounds. Cornwell and Goodrich (2010) say that in the UK, 'Observers at the initial rounds have also commented about how powerful it is to hear senior level clinicians and managers express their fears and concerns, the challenges they face and the reservations they sometimes feel when prescribing a particular course of action. Rounds provide the forum for staff to realise that they all, at times, struggle to make decisions and may in these situations be susceptible to self-doubt – and that these feelings do not necessarily disappear after years of experience or entry into management' (p. 12).

Adamson *et al.* (2009) say that it is clear that caring is the common denominator of what it actually means to be a nurse. However, they say that 'It is evident from nursing literature that there are difficulties in defining both caring itself and the idea of compassionate care' (p. 23). Adamson *et al.* (2009) say that Beauchamp and Childress (2009) refer to compassion as 'the prelude to caring, and caring has been described as the essence of nursing' (Adamson *et al.* 2009, p. 23). They describe the importance of the Leadership in Compassionate Care project, which is a joint initiative between Edinburgh

Napier University and NHS Lothian in Scotland. This project has focused on influencing nursing curriculum content (to ensure that compassionate care is a common theme for nursing and midwifery programmes), developing leadership skills in nurses so that they feel empowered to be key change agents in practice in relation to enhancing patient care, and has selected beacon wards to champion compassionate care. Having been to a conference led by staff involved with this project, we were very aware of how this approach was key to everything they believed in. They clearly practised what they preached; we have never been to such a caring conference, where students, educators, managers and practitioners demonstrated care of each other and of those who attended the conference.

In this section, we have focused on what contributes to an emotionally intelligent team culture because we believe that we need to use our emotional intelligence to work effectively as teams. We need to care about each other and the demands on us both personally and professionally. We need to create an environment where problems are addressed in a positive manner, and where everyone is encouraged to develop their leadership skills. High-quality care will be the norm when all quality strategies have compassion strongly embedded within them. Excellent care is not simply about the effectiveness of individual components of the caring process, it is about the whole patient journey from the first experience of care to the last. It includes whether parking is available to allow their loved ones to visit. It is about every episode of care and it is about continuity of care from one environment to another. It also involves listening to what is important to people in our care, and using their voice to influence our practice.

Dr Francis Peabody (1925) said that 'The secret of the care of the patient is in caring for the patient'. We need to remember that there is no magic solution to providing excellent care; however, it is essential that we do genuinely care for patients and clients, and that we care *about* them and not just *for* them. We also need to remember to care about each other and take a lead in ensuring that members of our teams feel cared about. To enhance care, we need to create a leadership culture (Kotter 1990) which focuses on the key components of high-quality care and encourages the development of leadership skills in all who work in our healthcare environments.

THOUGHTS FOR YOUR PRACTICE

- Do you work in an emotionally intelligent team culture?
- Do your leaders demonstrate emotionally intelligent team skills? Are they self-aware and socially aware, and are they able to manage themselves and their emotions? Do they have the ability to relate strongly with others? What could help them develop these skills further?
- Do you have emotionally intelligent team skills? What do you need to do to make these even better?
- Do you think that there are issues in relation to apathy, low morale and low levels of patient satisfaction in your practice area? How could these be addressed by a leader? Could you play a part in this?
- Do you think that there are sufficient opportunities to develop emotionally intelligent leadership skills? What do you think that you need to further develop yourself, and how are you going to achieve this development?
- How do you think that emotional intelligence affects the team ethos for individuals, your team leader and the wider organisation? Are there any historical factors in your team which could affect this?
- How do you think that emotional intelligence affects the attitudes and behaviour of your team? How could you increase the positive effect of this in your practice area?
- Are there any factors that affect interprofessional and interagency collaborative working in your team? Could these be influenced in any way, and if so, how?
- Do you think that there are any professional barriers that affect your ability to function effectively as a team? Are there any elements of the 'toxic team' in your practice area? If so, what role could you play in helping to reduce this problem?
- Think of a situation when there has been conflict in a team in which you have been working. How could you have used your own emotional intelligence to calm the situation down and to reduce the possibilities of the situation happening again?
- How could you use emotional intelligence to solve workplace issues? Can you easily identify issues which are task or relational based and internal or external in origin? What strategies could you try in the future to address these types of issues?
- Do you think that everyone in your practice area understands the importance

of addressing problems at an early stage? How could you help others to take a more active part in this?

- How could you adopt an emotionally intelligent leadership style to ensure that there is a positive team culture in which it is possible to learn as a team?
- Do you think that you work in an area where there is team and organisational learning? Do you feel empowered to learn as a team? How could this affect the quality of nursing care in your area?
- Do you think that there are ways in which the work-related emotional pressures in your area could be reduced? Try to think of some positive strategies which would help you and your colleagues feel more supported at work.
- Do you have any opportunities to reflect on and discuss the emotional impact of your caregiving? How could opportunities for these discussions be created or developed further? Could you take a lead in this, and if so, how?

SUMMARY

In this chapter, we have discussed the importance of the culture of the practice environment in providing excellent and compassionate care, and the import-ance of strong and effective leadership. As Kotter (1990) says, 'Just as we need more people to provide leadership in the complex organisations that domin-ate our world today, we also need more people to develop the cultures that will create that leadership. Institutionalising a leadership-centred culture is the ultimate act of leadership' (Kotter 1990, p. 96). While it is true that caring and empathetic nurses do not always make good managers or leaders, they do cre-ate the right cultural environment where patients remain a central focus. These nurses need to have motivational skills to help others to take a lead. They also need to develop a culture where constructive challenge is viewed positively so that high standards are maintained and enhanced. Everybody has the capacity to lead, but there need to be developmental opportunities to help people to realise their potential and to gain all the skills they require to motivate others to work towards the vision of excellent care.

Creating a compassionate culture in practice and taking a lead in this is challenging. There are many ways of contributing towards developing a posit-ive practice culture where excellent care is the norm. Every practice has its own emotional temperature and emotional climate. The importance of a positive approach and positive behaviour cannot be overestimated because positivity is contagious and will be mirrored in others' behaviour. Using approaches such as emotional touchpoints can help nurses to seek and respond to feedback from clients and patients in a positive way in order to enhance their care experience. The Senses Framework is also a way for patients and nurses to feel valued.

Inspirational, ethical and transformational leadership is key to enhancing practice, and having an inspirational vision is key to this. Leaders who are based with you as part of your team are easily accessible. Other leaders who operate at a more strategic level are more distant, but nevertheless have a clear part to play in developing policies that support excellent care. We all have a responsibility to help develop and nurture future leaders in nursing. There need to be effective role models for those who want to develop their leadership potential, and leaders and managers need to accept that through promoting high standards of care and high levels of staff motivation and performance, they are the role models.

Leaders and managers are key to creating a positive practice environment where staff feel motivated and satisfied with their roles and where people want to work. The approaches they take in their interactions with colleagues are key to this. Teams can be very diverse in their experience, expectations, ages, genders and cultural norms, and this can be a real strength. However, it can also cause friction points which need to be resolved. It is important to create stable teams where staff have specific roles and feel valued for their expertise and supported in their development; a caring environment such as this has a real impact on recruitment and retention. A good nurse leader has clear vision, ensures competent, safe and evidence-based care, is an effective communicator and creates a positive team culture and climate.

The development of an emotionally intelligent team culture is key to a positive practice environment. Relational leadership is essential through the building and maintaining of relationships in the workplace. There are clear correlations between emotional intelligence and leadership, with clear links to patient satisfaction and quality of care. Nurses need to manage their emotions when they are at work in order to be effective; when there is conflict in a team, this is not always the case. Nurses need to be self-aware, have high self-regard, be assertive, be independent, manage their stress and regulate themselves in order to achieve their potential. All of these are important attributes of emotionally intelligent practitioners, leaders and teams. A strong team ethos, with appropriate attitudes and behaviour, and strong interprofessional and interagency collaboration, is the antithesis of a 'toxic team' situation where emotionally intelligent teamworking is severely lacking. Where conflict and problems do exist, they need to be addressed as quickly as possible, identifying whether the problems are task or relationship orientated and involve internal or external factors. Otherwise these issues can severely impact on a team's intelligence and ability to learn together. Having opportunities to reflect on the stresses of the situations that arise within nursing practice can be key to high staff morale, motivation and retention rates, and to low degrees of staff sickness, stress and emotional burnout, and thereby promote excellent nursing care.

In the next chapter, we discuss the positive individual attitudinal attributes that practitioners and leaders of care need to have in order to ensure that practice is of a high quality in these dynamic and challenging times.

REFERENCES

Abraham A. *Care and compassion? Report of the Health Service Ombudsman on ten investigations into NHS care of older people.* London: Stationery Office; 2011.

AbuAlRub R, Al-Zaru I. Job stress, recognition, job performance and intention to stay at work among Jordanian hospital nurses. *J Nurs Manag.* 2008; **16**(3): 227–36.

Adamson E, King L, Moody J, *et al.* Developing a nursing education project in partnership: leadership in compassionate care. *Nurs Times.* 2009; **105**(35): 23–6.

Akerjordet K, Severinsson E. Emotionally intelligent nurse leadership: a literature review study. *J Nurs Manag.* 2008; **16**(5): 565–77.

Alimo-Metcalfe B, Alban-Metcalfe J. More (good) leaders for the public sector. *Int J Public Sect Manag.* 2006; **19**(4): 293–315.

Ashton S. Using compliments to measure quality. *Nurs Times.* 2011; **107**(7): 14–15.

Beauchamp T, Childress J. *Principles of Biomedical Ethics.* Oxford: Oxford University Press; 2009.

Braynion P. Power and leadership. *J Health Organ Manag.* 2004; **18**(6): 447–63.

Burnham D. *Power Is Still the Great Motivator – With a Difference!* 2007. www.burn hamrosen.com/articles/power_is_still.pdf (accessed 11 December 2011).

Chambers C, Ryder E. *Compassion and Caring in Nursing.* Oxford: Radcliffe Publishing; 2009.

Cook M. The renaissance of clinical leadership. *Int Nurs Rev.* 2001; **48**(1): 38–46.

Cornwell J. Evidence is piling up that nurse leaders who really care about patients must pay attention to how their staff feel about work. *Nurs Times.* 2010; **106**(10): 8–9.

Cornwell J, Goodrich J. Supporting staff to deliver compassionate care using Schwartz Center Rounds: a UK pilot. *Nurs Times.* 2010; **106**(5): 10–12.

Covey S. *The 8th Habit: from effectiveness to greatness.* New York: Simon and Schuster; 2006.

Cummings G, Hayduk L, Estabrooks C. Mitigating the impact of hospital restructuring on nurses. *Nurs Res.* 2005; **54**(1): 2–12.

Cummings G, Olson K, Hayduk L, *et al.* The relationship between nursing leadership and nurses' job satisfaction in Canadian oncology work environments. *J Nurs Manag.* 2008; **16**(5): 508–18.

De Cooman R, De Gieter S, Pepermans R, *et al.* Freshmen in nursing: job motives and work values of a new generation. *J Nurs Manag.* 2008; **16**(1): 56–64.

Department of Health. *NHS Health and Well-Being Review: interim report.* London: Stationery Office; 2009.

Dewar B, Mackay R, Smith S, *et al.* Use of emotional touchpoints as a method of tapping into the experience of receiving compassionate care in a hospital setting. *J Res Nurs.* 2010; **15**(1): 29–41.

Dewar B, Ogilvie H. Using *All about Me* booklet to improve relationship centred care: briefing. *NHS Lothian and Edinburgh Napier University Inaugural International Conference on Compassionate Care.* 2010 Jun 9–11; Edinburgh.

Farag A, Tullai-McGuiness S, Anthony M. Nurses' perception of their manager's leadership style and unit climate: are there generational differences? *J Nurs Manag.* 2009; **17**(1): 26–34.

Firth-Cozens J, Cornwell J. *The Point of Care: enabling compassionate care in acute hospital settings.* London: King's Fund; 2009.

Francis R. *Independent inquiry into care provided by Mid Staffordshire NHS Foundation Trust January 2005–March 2009.* Volume 1. London: Stationery Office; 2010.

Freedman J. *At the Heart of Leadership: how to get results with emotional intelligence.* Freedom, CA: Six Seconds Emotional Intelligence Press; 2007.

Gillon R. Philosophical medical ethics. 1994. In: Palfrey C, Thomas P, Phillips C. Health services management: what are the ethical dimensions? *Int J Public Sect Manag.* 2006; **19**(1): 57–66.

Goleman D, Boyatzis R, McKee A. *The New Leaders: transforming the art of leadership into the science of results.* London: Sphere; 2002.

Goodman Research Group. *Schwartz Center Rounds Evaluation Report.* Cambridge, MA: Goodman Research Group; 2008.

Govier I, Nash S. Examining transformational approaches to effective leadership in healthcare settings. *Nurs Times.* 2009; **105**(18): 24–7.

Groves K, McEnrue M, Shen W. Developing and measuring the emotional intelligence of leaders. *J Manag Dev.* 2008; **27**(2): 225–50.

Hemmelgarn A, Glisson C, James L. Organisational culture and climate: implications for services and interventions research. *Clin Psychol Sci Prac.* 2006; **13**(1): 73–89.

Hill S. Team leadership. In: Northouse P. *Leadership: theory and practice.* London: Sage Publications; 2007.

Kennedy R. How do we get the managers we need and the leaders we want? A personal view. *J Nurs Manag.* 2008; **16**(8): 942–5.

Kotter J. What leaders really do. *Harvard Business Review.* 1990 May–June; 103–11.

Kuokkanen L, Suominen T, Rankinen S, *et al.* Organisational change and work-related empowerment. *J Nurs Manag.* 2007; **15**(5): 500–7.

Lees L. Managers must support nurses to boost their commitment to care. *Nurs Times.* 2009; **105**(48): 9.

Lucas V, Laschinger H, Wong C. The impact of emotional intelligent leadership on staff nurse empowerment: the moderating effect of span of control. *J Nurs Manag.* 2008; **16**(8): 964–73.

Maben J, Latter S, Clark JM. The sustainability of ideals, values and the nursing mandate: evidence from a longitudinal qualitative study. *Nurs Inq.* 2007; **14**(2): 99–113.

McClelland D, Burnham D. Power is the great motivator. *Harvard Business Review.* 1995 Jan–Feb; 126–39.

McClelland D. Business drive and national achievement. *Harvard Business Review.* 1962 Jul–Aug; 99–112.

McGregor D. *The Human Side of Enterprise: annotated edition.* New York, NY: McGraw-Hill; 2006.

McNamara C. *Organizational Culture.* Minneapolis, MN: Authenticity Consulting; 2000. Available at: http://managementhelp.org/organizations/culture.htm (accessed 17 December 2011).

Martin R. How successful leaders think. *Harvard Business Review.* 2007; **85**(6): 60–7.

Masterson A, Gough P. Adaptable leaders are crucial to the new NHS. *Nurs Times.* 2010; **106**(34): 23.

Nash S, Govier I. Effective team leadership: techniques that nurses can use to improve teamworking. *Nurs Times.* 2009; **105**(19): 22–4.

Nicholls J. The heart, head and hands of transforming leadership. *Leadership Organis Dev J.* 1994; **15**(6): 8–15.

Nolan Committee. Standards in public life. 1995. In: Palfrey C, Thomas P, Phillips C. Health services management: what are the ethical dimensions? *Int J Public Sect Manag.* 2006; **19**(1): 57–66.

Nolan M, Brown J, Davies S, *et al. The Senses Framework: improving care for older people through a relationship-centred approach.* Sheffield: University of Sheffield; 2006.

Northouse P. *Introduction to Leadership: concepts and practice.* London: Sage Publications; 2009.

Paetzold R, Dipboye R, Elsbach K. A new look at stigmatization in and of organisations. *Acad Manag Rev.* 2008; **33**(1): 186–93.

Palfrey C, Thomas P, Phillips C. Health services management: what are the ethical dimensions? *Int J Pub Sect Manag.* 2006; **19**(1): 57–66.

Park J, Kim T. Do types of organisational culture matter in nurse job satisfaction and turnover intention? *Leadersh Health Serv (Bradf Engl).* 2009; **22**(1): 20–38.

Peabody F. www.art-of-patient-care.com 1925; (accessed 13 January 2012).

Pilgrim D, Sheaff R. Can learning organisations survive in the newer NHS? *Implement Sci.* 2006; **1**: 27. Available at: www.implementationscience.com/content/1/1/27 (accessed 11 December 2011).

Pillay R. Retention strategies for professional nurses in South Africa. *Leadersh Health Serv (Bradf Engl).* 2009; **22**(1): 39–57.

Ritter D. The relationship between healthy work environments and retention of nurses in a hospital setting. *J Nurs Manag.* 2011; **19**(1): 27–32.

Robbins H, Finley M. *Why Teams Don't Work.* London: Texere; 2000.

Ross F. Poor organisational cultures erode compassionate care. *Nurs Times.* 2010; **106**(33): 27.

Santry C. Nurse leadership severely lacking. *Nurs Times.* 2011; **107**(7): 2–3.

Schwartz K. A patient's story. *The Boston Globe Magazine*. 1995 Jul 16. Available at: www.theschwartzcenter.org/ViewPage.aspx?pageId=50 (accessed 11 December 2011).

Senge P. The fifth discipline: the art and practice of the learning organisation. 1990. In: Smith M. *Peter Senge and the Learning Organisation*. 2001 (last update 1 Dec 2011). Available at: www.infed.org/thinkers/senge.htm (accessed 11 December 2011).

Smith M. *Peter Senge and the Learning Organisation*. 2001 (last update 1 Dec 2011). Available at: www.infed.org/thinkers/senge.htm (accessed 11 December 2011).

Sparrow T, Knight A. *Applied EI: the importance of attitudes in developing emotional intelligence*. Chichester: John Wiley & Sons; 2006.

St Pierre I, Holmes D. Managing nurses through disciplinary power: a Foucauldian analysis of workplace violence. *J Nurs Manag*. 2008; **16**(3): 352–9.

Stubbs Koman E, Wolff S. Emotional intelligence competencies in the team and team leader: a multi-level examination of the impact of emotional intelligence on team performance. *J Manag Dev*. 2008; **27**(1): 55–75.

Swearingen S, Liberman A. Nursing generations: an expanded look at the emergence of conflict and its resolution. *Health Care Manag*. 2004; **23**(1): 54–64.

Tomey AM. Nursing leadership and management effects work environments. *J Nurs Manag*. 2009; **17**: 15–25.

Wang C, Ahmed P. Organisational learning: a critical review. *The Learning Organisation*. 2003; **10**(1): 8–18.

Wedderburn Tate C. *Leadership in Nursing*. London: Churchill Livingstone; 1999.

Westwood C. *How to Succeed as a Nurse Leader*. Available at: www.nursingtimes.net/forums-blogs-ideas-debate/your-career/the-happy-nurse/how-to-suceed-as-a-nurse-leader/5012783.article (accessed 11 December 2011).

White M. *Creating a Positive Emotional Temperature*. 2008. Available at: www.management-issues.com/2008/2/12/opinion/creating-a-positive-emotional-temperature.asp (accessed 11 December 2011).

Wong C, Cummings G. The relationship between nursing leadership and patient outcomes: a systematic review. *J Nurs Manag*. 2007; **15**(5): 508–21.

www.mater.org.au/Home/About/Mission-Vision-and-Values

www.nhsleadershipqualities.nhs.uk (2006) and revised www.nhsleadership.org.uk/framework.asp (2011).

www.mindtools.com/pages/article/newTMC_5W.htm

www.theschwartzcenter.org

CHAPTER 4

Nurse attitude – the heart of compassionate care

OVERVIEW OF THE CHAPTER

We have discussed the importance of providing excellent compassionate nursing care throughout the previous chapters, particularly in relation to how nurses can, and should, take the lead in the care that is carried out in their practice areas. In our first book on compassion and caring in nursing (Chambers and Ryder 2009), we identified three potential challenges to compassionate care, namely, resourcing and the culture of the nursing environment, which we have already discussed in Chapter 2 and Chapter 3 of this book, and the individual nurse attitude, which we will discuss in this chapter. We see individual nurse attitude as the most crucial challenge in relation to both individual standards of practice and the ability to lead practice forward. If a nurse believes strongly in the need for patients and clients to receive good care, then they will not tolerate substandard care in themselves or others and will want to bring about change. If they feel that on any given day care could have been better, they will reflect on the particular circumstances of that day and try to develop ways of addressing the issues that caused the problems, because these issues are unlikely to have happened in isolation. Such nurses will not blame inadequate resourcing as the total reason for ongoing poor care, or excuse themselves on the grounds that nobody else was able to be compassionate and caring either. They will be thinking as leaders, in terms of enhancing care and believing that they can make a difference within their practice area.

The NHS Leadership Qualities Framework (2006) and the NHS Leadership Framework (2011), as already discussed in Chapter 2, clearly identify the importance of setting direction and personal qualities in order to deliver the service. Personal qualities are key components of healthcare leadership. In this chapter, we focus on the personal qualities of a leader in practice. In the NHS Leadership Qualities Framework (2006), these are identified as being:

➤ self-belief
➤ self-awareness
➤ self-management
➤ drive for improvement
➤ personal integrity.

Leaders who have these personal qualities have personal confidence and want to shape the way that things are carried out. They know their strengths and limitations, can pace themselves and can manage their own behaviour. They also constantly want to improve the service, give of their best, achieve their potential and help others achieve theirs. In the redeveloped NHS Leadership framework (www.nhsleadership.org.uk), personal qualities remain key to delivering the required service, along with setting direction, improving and managing services and working with others. These are all essential components of creating a vision and delivering an appropriate strategy for care in any practice environment.

An expert nurse is not necessarily one who knows about complex technology, though this can be the case; an expert nurse is one who knows how to make someone feel cared about in terms of providing fundamental care (Santry 2010), and who tries to find out what a client enjoys or is distressed by. As Jopson (2010) says, it can be the small things in life that make the most difference to someone's experience, and he gives examples of one of his clients having the opportunity to simply enjoy the sunshine and of another savouring an ice cream. Newton (2010) also agrees with this point and says that when someone is distressed or unwell, the most important element of their care, as far as they are concerned, is being cared for with compassion. She stresses the importance of good role-modelling in helping more junior members of staff to understand the importance of this, and to emulate this level of compassion.

Nicholson *et al.* (2010a, 2010b, 2010c) write about the importance of practical interventions in relation to the Dignity in Care project in the UK. This project involves getting to know the person behind the patient, or the person behind the nurse, by focusing on 'seeing who I am', 'connecting with me' and 'involving me'. This enables enhanced communication where patients and nurses can value each other, and members of the team can work together to enhance care. Shared decision making with patients and all members of the team can then be actively facilitated, and person-centred care can become more of a reality than is often the case in very rushed clinical environments. Radcliffe (2010) asks why nurses are sometimes rude: is it because they are thoughtless and have forgotten how important good communication is, or because they are having a bad day? Or is it because they are subconsciously choosing to be rude, maybe because they are feeling undervalued themselves? As he says (p. 28), 'It's a worrying choice, isn't it? The idea that some nurses are lacking in basic communication skills or are choosing to be rude or aggressive. Either way, it needs to be addressed. Communication is the heart of nursing; if that stops beating, we are really in trouble.' Rowan (2009) reiterates this point in her student nurse blog when she discusses her experience of being a patient. She differentiates between 'grumpy nurse', 'happy nurse', 'super nurse' and 'nice nurse', all of whom had different ways of communicating. 'Grumpy nurse' did not smile or introduce herself, and increased her (Rowan's) level of stress, whereas the others all did, and by doing so helped her relax and trust them. As she says, 'Communication, compassion and trust are vital elements of nursing, but the ability to communicate is perhaps the most important' (Rowan 2009).

Nicholson *et al.* (2010b) suggest that a way of assessing the quality of communication in different interactions could be through the use of the shortened quality of interaction schedule (SQUIS) stop, look, listen observation tool (Ashburner *et al.* 2004). The different interactions that SQUIS focuses on are:

> positive social interaction (PS) – empathetic, connecting with the person
> basic care interaction (BC) – gets the task accomplished
> neutral interaction (N) – brief and indifferent
> negative interaction (N–) – ignores, patronises or is rude.

In Nicholson *et al.*'s work (2010b), the quality of communication was discussed as a ward team focusing on good and compassionate communication to try to think about processes which could reduce or eliminate poorer ways of communicating.

The importance of taking a lead on compassionate communication is a central tenet of the personal qualities highlighted in the NHS Leadership Qualities Framework (2006), the NHS Leadership Framework (2011) and in all the writing on emotional intelligence. Radcliffe (2010) says that nurses tend to meet people at times of difficulty: when the person or a loved one is ill and in need of care. He asks how we can create environments where nurses can be emotionally excellent or emotionally brilliant. Are they supported and enabled to be these types of practitioners or are they left to burn themselves out? It is the role of a leader to ensure that they empower and support other nurses to achieve their potential and to maximise the opportunities for excellent care.

In this chapter, we discuss the positive leadership attitudes that ensure this is the case. It is important to understand what the attributes of a leader actually are and how we can enhance our personal effectiveness as leaders. We all need to see it as our own personal mission to bring about positive change and rediscover how to be most effective as leaders who ensure that nursing practice is of the highest level possible.

KEY THEME ONE – TAKING THE LEAD IN EXCELLENT COMPASSIONATE NURSING CARE

CASE STUDY 4.1

Lizzy, a school nurse, had been running the 'drop-in' at the local secondary school for the whole term. The room was far from ideal, but finding a room at all in the busy school environment was always a challenge. The noise from outside was variable, but could be intrusive during conversations when a student was talking quietly. On the other hand, it meant that nothing could be overheard from outside. A more pressing problem was that the room contained a store cupboard which members of staff often needed to access. Despite a notice on the door asking for no interruptions, individuals seemed not to think that this applied to them.

This particular day, Lizzy was sitting writing notes when there was a tentative knock on the door. A rather timid-looking boy came into the room looking very embarrassed, and he blushed as soon as she made eye contact. She immediately smiled at him and introduced herself, and he said that his name was Zack. Lizzy started to make social conversation to put him at ease. She asked Zack what he enjoyed doing in his spare time. He said that he enjoyed going to the local youth group, where they were able to do a range of activities. He started fidgeting at this point and stopped making eye contact with her. She sensed his distress and the fact that he did not know how to tell her what he wanted to say. Lizzy asked him how old he was, and he replied that he was 12, and she asked him who he spent most time with while he was there. He blurted out the name Jon and then blushed again and looked away. Lizzy started gently probing by asking questions, and Zack eventually revealed that Jon was a leader at the club, was in his 30s and had started to touch Zack in a way that made him feel uncomfortable. Lizzy immediately felt a real sense of anger that someone who was in a responsible position in a youth group could cause such distress in a 12-year-old. Zack clearly respected and admired Jon and did not want to believe that he was behaving inappropriately, and he was blaming himself for what had taken place.

Just as Zack was beginning to make eye contact again with Lizzy, and she could sense that he was starting to trust her, a member of staff knocked on the door, came in without waiting for a response and announced that he just needed to get a book from the cupboard. Lizzy saw Zack flinch, shrink against the wall and try to hide his tears. She went to meet the member of staff and said very calmly – with clear eye contact – that she needed to have the room for the next 20 minutes, and he appeared to understand her unspoken message and immediately left the room.

Lizzy turned back to Zack, smiled at him again and asked him if he was comfortable with her sitting with her back against the door so that they could not be interrupted again, because there was no lock for the door. He turned to face where she was now sitting, seemed to be relieved and started to speak again.

How do you further develop positive leadership attributes to enhance nursing care?

Nursing does not always take place in a hospital, and the way in which public health, mental health or learning disability nurses interact with clients can be very different. Conversations can take place in a range of different environments where circumstances can be far from ideal. Visits that take place in the home or schools can be challenging in terms of privacy, and the environment can have a strong negative impact on communication skills and strategies. Lizzy was trying to communicate with Zack in difficult circumstances about difficult issues after having only just met him. This was bound to very challenging for her and needed an advanced level of communication skill to make the interchange therapeutic and effective. Eye contact was very important, and when Zack was at his most embarrassed he avoided it. However, Lizzy persevered, and he eventually started to look at her again. When the staff member interrupted this delicate situation, she did not overreact, but stayed calm and conveyed a strong message with her eyes that she hoped he would understand, and it worked well. Many nurses have become very skilled at communicating messages and meaning without words, with both patients and carers and with colleagues. Rungapadiachy (1999) says that eye contact tends to lessen when we feel that something is not acceptable. Therefore, Lizzy might have maintained appropriate eye contact with Zack, but could have been so irritated by the interruption that she might not have made eye contact with the teacher. However, by doing so, she managed to help him to understand the urgency of her message without alienating him.

Being present when someone chooses to self-disclose is a very privileged position to be in. Self-disclosure, according to Rungapadiachy (1999), is an incremental process where non-disclosure moves into disclosure, although this may be only partial disclosure. How much one chooses to disclose can be clearly related to the level of trust and communication skill displayed by the other person.

Lizzy had a high level of self-awareness; she understood the emotions and priorities of others. She knew that she could easily break the fragile initial level of trust that was building up between herself and Zack. However, she needed to help the staff member to understand the situation without explaining the details to him, and in a way that maintained a cordial professional relationship.

She had to regulate her own emotions in this difficult situation. She was angry about the situation that Zack was in, and she was also concerned about the interruption at such a sensitive time. It would have been easy to have reacted in a negative manner towards the member of staff who was trying to enter the room.

Self-awareness and the management of emotions are important components of emotional intelligence (Chapman 2001), which in itself is a key attribute of positive leadership. Goleman *et al.* (2002) say that resonant leaders create enthusiastic and cohesive teams where there is cooperation and trust, and 'resonance comes naturally to emotionally intelligent leaders' (p. 25). So in demonstrating self-awareness, self-management, social awareness and relationship management, Lizzy was demonstrating her skills as a resonant, emotionally intelligent leader. Her immediate focus was on Zack, but she was also aware of the importance of managing her own behaviour and emotions, so that her relationship with other members of staff was not damaged. She needed to be empathetic towards both Zack and the teacher, whose priorities were very different at that point. The teacher needed to get some books for the next class, but although he would have been very concerned for Zack's well-being, he was not aware of the sensitive nature of the discussion. Lizzy was able to behave in a way that was acceptable to both parties by demonstrating relationship management and resonant leadership. In a Canadian study, Cummings *et al.* (2005) say that 'Empathetic leaders are attuned to a wide range of emotional signals, allowing them to sense the felt, but unspoken, emotions in another person or group' (p. 3). So it could be said that the teacher was also demonstrating resonant emotionally intelligent leadership by understanding Lizzy's unspoken message. Cummings *et al.* (2005) also say that nurses working for resonant leaders suffer less emotional ill health, experience greater job satisfaction and collaborate better with others from different professions. This was true in the relationship between Lizzy and the teacher. Dissonant leaders tend to focus more on pace of work and telling people what to do, and these are occasionally necessary, but as Goleman *et al.* (2002) say, they need to be used sparingly. Resonant leaders demonstrate:

➤ self-awareness
  — emotional self-awareness
  — accurate self-assessment
  — self-confidence
➤ self-management
  — self-control
  — transparency
  — adaptability
  — achievement
  — initiative
  — optimism
➤ social awareness
  — empathy
  — organisational awareness
  — service
➤ relationship management
  — inspiration
  — influence
  — developing others
  — change catalyst
  — conflict management
  — teamwork and collaboration. (Goleman *et al.* 2002, Appendix B)

Lizzy's approach in this difficult situation used her self-awareness, self-regulation and social awareness to avoid conflict and to keep alive a collaborative approach with other professionals. By demonstrating that she was motivated and empathetic, Lizzy conveyed to Zack that she had time for him. In contrast, Santry (2010) describes how nurses often adopt body language that discourages people from disclosing their fears and concerns. It is really important that nurses do not show signs of distraction when communicating with others, and they need to keep re-evaluating their communication skills, however experienced they are.

Horton-Deutsch and Sherwood (2008) emphasise the importance of emotional competence in relation to nurse leadership, and how reflection can be a useful tool in helping to prepare emotionally capable leaders. Lizzy demonstrated her emotional intelligence as a practitioner and a leader in this scenario. She was able to 'reflect in action', as well as 'reflect on action' (Schon 1987), so that she could adapt her reactions and behaviour at the time. This enabled her to focus on the needs of both Zack and the staff member during the interaction. Had she been unable to do so, her relationship with both Zack and the teacher might have weakened, both then and in the future, and later she might have reflected on how she could have acted differently.

In our first book on compassion and caring in nursing (Chambers and Ryder 2009), we highlighted the importance of nurses aiming for more than emotional intelligence in their nursing and client-focused care. Goleman (1996) talks about 'emotional brilliance' and we said how those in our care need us to be at our absolute best; they need to experience our emotional brilliance. As nurse leaders, we need also to demonstrate emotional brilliance in our relationships with colleagues, because it is so easy for team relationships to deteriorate and for members of staff to become resentful, demotivated and disempowered. Nursing is a stressful environment where a great deal is expected of us, and if we do not make it supportive and energising then stressed members of staff will become even more vulnerable, and nobody will be able to give of their best. Goleman (1996) says that 'If the test of social skill is the ability to calm distressing emotions in others, then handling someone at the peak of rage is perhaps the ultimate measure of mastery' (p. 124). Using empathy to help that person focus on alternative ways of thinking can be an effective way to defuse anger. Nobody was angry in the case study, but due to heightened emotions they could easily have become so. The teacher could have thought that his need to access learning materials before a class was not being taken seriously, and Zack could have felt that his situation was not being taken seriously either, or he could have decided to stop talking at that point. Lizzy could have become angry at the interruption and her inability to maintain focus on Zack's issues; her emotional brilliance was definitely needed.

The importance of empathy in understanding your own emotions, as well as those of others, cannot be underestimated in relation to emotional intelligence. Goleman (1996) cites Sifneos (1972) and uses the term 'alexithymic' to describe people who do have feelings but do not understand them and cannot put them into words. Alexythmics are completely without emotional intelligence because they lack self-awareness, which requires knowing what they feel. By lacking empathy, they also lack insight, and as Goleman (1996) says, they are 'emotionally tone deaf' (p. 96). People who are the antithesis of emotionally intelligent can cause great problems in the work environment due to their lack of understanding of the feelings of others, and they do not make good leaders for the same reason. Chapman (2001) has summarised Hein's (1996) work on the 10 habits of emotionally intelligent people who:

➤ label their feelings, rather than labelling people or situations
➤ distinguish between thoughts and feelings
➤ take responsibility for their feelings
➤ use their emotions to help make decisions
➤ show respect for others' feelings
➤ feel energised, not angry
➤ validate others' feelings
➤ practise getting a positive value from their negative emotions
➤ do not advise, command, control, criticise, blame or judge others
➤ avoid people who invalidate them or don't respect their feelings (Chapman 2001, p. 88).

Lizzy did her best to behave in this manner in her sensitive encounter with Zack. She used all her communication skills as well as her positive personality. Peterson and Seligman (2004) wrote a key text on character strengths and virtues in which they identified six positive character traits that are key to positive psychology. Positive psychology focuses on the strength of individuals to help them achieve their highest potential. It aims at promoting the best things in life and repairing the worst, in order to help alleviate distress in those who are experiencing it. According to Peterson and Seligman (2004), the six main character strengths are:

➤ wisdom and knowledge – creativity, curiosity, open-mindedness, love of learning, perspective
➤ courage – bravery, persistence, integrity, vitality
➤ humanity – love, kindness (compassion), social intelligence (emotional and personal intelligence)
➤ justice – citizenship (social responsibility), fairness, leadership
➤ temperance – forgiveness and mercy, humility and modesty, prudence, self-regulation
➤ transcendence – appreciation of beauty and excellence, gratitude, hope (optimism and future orientation), humour, spirituality (religiousness, faith and purpose).

Lizzy clearly demonstrated wisdom in that she had a clear understanding of everyone's perspectives in this situation, coupled with knowledge of how crucial the experience was for Zack's future well-being and what could have a negative effect on his ability to talk with her. She also demonstrated persistence and integrity (courage) in redirecting the conversation back to Zack after the interruption. She understood the need to take a lead (justice), and demonstrated temperance by her self-regulation when she was understandably concerned about the interruption at a crucial point in the discussion. To some extent, transcendence could be seen in Lizzy's sense of purpose and her hope that Zack's situation could improve if he had the advice that he needed. However, Lizzy's particular strength in this situation was most clearly demonstrated in her humanity because she genuinely cared about Zack, and her social intelligence was clear in her personal and emotional intelligence. In addition, she demonstrated kindness, which Peterson and Seligman (2004) state includes generosity, nurturance, care, compassion, altruistic love and 'niceness'.

As practitioners and leaders, we all need to be aware of how to use our positivity and our personal positive psychological skills in order to take a lead in enhancing practice development. However, to be able to take a lead in difficult situations, it is essential to have an internal locus of control (Rotter 1966), and feel that some measure of control lies within you. You also need to have some degree of self-efficacy, that is, a sense of feeling personally effective in determining what happens around you. Nurses and other practitioners can feel a sense of 'learned helplessness' (Seligman 1975) if this is not the case, because they feel that nothing they do makes any difference. Lizzy clearly felt that she had some control over the circumstances of her interaction with Zack. Her innate internal locus of control and self-efficacy meant that she was able to influence the situation on Zack's behalf and so minimise the effect of the teacher's interruption. Lizzy must have felt stressed by the situation that had arisen because she wanted to help Zack as much as she could, and she could sense his vulnerability without fully knowing its basis. Cassidy (1999) says that what makes a stressor stressful is the extent of control and predictability someone has in any given situation. We need to be able to predict outcomes in order to feel in control. The fact that neither Zack nor Lizzy could be sure of their conversation being undisturbed caused additional stress for both of them. This is a common situation for many nurses, in that privacy and undisturbed time with patients and clients can be very difficult to achieve. It is important that they take steps to ensure that important discussions can be allowed to continue without interruption, whether they be with patients, clients or colleagues. Misunderstandings and feelings of being undervalued can result from practitioners being disturbed in their discussions with managers, or nurses being interrupted in their care and conversations with people in their care. Rungapadiachy (2008) interestingly says that you do not need to *exercise* that control in order to be effective – simply knowing it is there is empowering. He goes on to say that control does not need to be real; perceived control can be as effective as actual control (Rungapadiachy 2008). This is an interesting point, and as leaders in practice we need to ensure that colleagues and patients or clients feel that they have some degree of control, even if it is limited by external factors or organisational pressures. This will have a positive effect on their self-esteem and self-concept, and they will be more effective in their lives and their work environments as a result.

Lizzy clearly felt some degree of control, even though this was only one of the many schools she visited, and she did not know this member of staff well. She had a positive self-image and was personally and professionally competent and confident. Rungapadiachy (2008) discusses the importance of self-concept and identifies different levels of self-concept: physical (for example body image), social (autonomy, role, status, interactions), emotional (control over feelings) and intellectual (use of language, previous experiences and problem-solving ability). Lizzy clearly had a positive self-concept in all these areas and was able to stay calm, problem-solve and maintain her relationship with both Zack and the teacher – a demonstration of the high level of skill that she was using.

Furnham (2008) says that there are different 'intelligences' that we use in our everyday lives. These include:

➤ intelligence quotient (IQ) – information processing, a good memory and the ability to learn
➤ technical/operational quotient (TQ) – ability to manage ideas and projects, understand relevant technology and generally get things done
➤ motivational quotient (MQ) – desire to achieve, lead and succeed
➤ experience quotient (XQ) – quantity and quality of experience
➤ people quotient (PQ) – self-awareness and self-management of motives, emotions and actions and their effect on others
➤ learning quotient (LQ) – ability to think, manage and solve problems in different ways (Furnham 2008, pp. 9–10).

We would add another intelligence:
➤ cultural quotient (CQ) – ability to adapt to new cultural contexts (Earley and Ang 2003, cited in Berry *et al.* 2011) and to acquire new ways of acting to meet new demands (Gudykunst and Hammer 1983, cited in Berry *et al.* 2011).

Lizzy clearly was able to use all these forms of intelligence in her nursing role. She was intellectually capable of understanding the importance of the conversation with Zack, and operationally intelligent in trying to ensure that it took place. She was motivationally intelligent in making sure that she took a lead in making it happen. She was experientially intelligent, so she understood the potential effect of the interruption on Jack, and her people quotient was high, so she managed her emotions in order to maintain effective relationships with both Zack and the teacher. She also had high learning quotient skills, so she could think, adapt and problem-solve quickly to minimise the impact of the interruption.

We added cultural intelligence, because as we said in the previous chapter, the culture of the practice environment has a large impact on the care that takes place. This skill enabled Lizzy to adapt to new demands in different environments. As nurses, we need to use all our intelligence as well as our clinical expertise in order to achieve maximum benefit for the patient or client.

Furnham (2008) goes on to discuss emotional intelligences at work in the form of personal competencies:

➤ self-awareness – emotional self-awareness, accurate self-assessment, self-confidence
➤ self-regulation – self-control, trustworthiness, conscientiousness, adaptability, innovation
➤ motivation – achievement drive, commitment, initiative, optimism
➤ empathy – understanding and developing others, service orientation, cultivating opportunities through different kinds of people, political awareness
➤ social skills – influence, communication, conflict management, leadership, change catalyst, building relationships, collaboration and cooperation, team capabilities (Furnham 2008, pp. 16–17).

It is important that as nurses, we use all the emotional intelligences that we have in order to become 'emotionally brilliant' (Goleman 1996). Lizzy demonstrated clearly her ability to be self-aware, self-regulated and to be motivated and empathetic. She used all her social skills to avoid alienating or discouraging both parties and to maintain strong relationships with her colleague and Zack.

These are all positive attributes that are used consistently by experienced and sensitive nurses to lead practice forward and to enhance their relationships with people in their care.

THOUGHTS FOR YOUR PRACTICE

- How could you enhance your focus on hidden messages (messages and meaning without words) in your communication with others?
- How do you ensure that you create opportunities for people to disclose their personal situations if they want to?
- Think of a recent practice situation and use this to develop your thinking in relation to how you could use your emotional intelligence to greater effect.
- Identify leaders in your practice area and analyse what aspects of their personalities make them more resonant or dissonant leaders. How can you become more of a resonant leader in your relationships with others?
- Identify times when you have been able to reflect in action. Also, think of times when you gained different perspectives by reflecting on action after the event.
- In what way could you become more emotionally brilliant? What strategies do you need to use in order to make sure that you focus on this to a greater extent?
- Have you ever worked with people who have alexithymic characteristics? If so, how do you think that you could build an effective working relationship with them?
- Think about your personality. What are your most positive psychological traits? What areas could you further develop in order to feel more positive in life?
- How could you increase the degree of control and predictability in your working environment for yourself and others?
- How could you build on different aspects of your self-concept, and how could you enhance these in others?
- Identify ways in which you use different intelligences in your practice. Try to think of ways in which you can develop areas which you tend to use less frequently.
- Look at the different personal competencies of emotional intelligence and identify which areas you want to focus on to increase your level of emotional intelligence in practice.

ONGOING PRACTICE – DISCUSSION ONE

Lizzy continued to make eye contact with Zack – she wanted to show him how interested she was in what he had to say. Zack looked unsettled and kept looking at the door as if he thought that someone else might come in at any minute. Lizzy said that she could see he was concerned about privacy and asked him what would make him feel more comfortable and help him feel more secure in the knowledge that nobody else would overhear what he wanted to discuss with her. He said that he wanted to be sure nobody else could come into the room without permission. Lizzy asked him what they could do that would reassure him about this. Zack felt that writing a note on the door would give a strong message that this was a private discussion, but Lizzy replied that a note was already there. Zack said that he did not want to lock the door, even if there was a key, but he suggested that he sat on a chair against the door so that nobody could come in without banging into his chair first. He said this would give him warning and allow him time to collect himself before they saw that he was distressed. Lizzy agreed that this was a good idea. She had not suggested that she sat there herself because she did not want him to feel trapped. She did not feel threatened by him in any way, and therefore had no concerns about feeling trapped herself. Zack also suggested that she could discuss the importance of privacy with the head teacher. She agreed to do this, and Zack visibly relaxed and continued to talk about what had been happening when he saw Jon on his own.

How can you enhance your personal effectiveness as a leader?

We have discussed how we can use our emotional intelligences and personal attributes in a positive way to enhance our leadership. However, we need to think about how we can be as effective as possible in order to take a lead on enhancing excellent and compassionate care.

Thompson (2009) highlights the importance of managing ourselves effectively in relation to working with others. Self-awareness is key, because otherwise we do not know what the impact of what we say and do has on others around us. Self-management involves managing our time and our stress effectively. Unfortunately, many practitioners and managers do not do this and constantly disappoint others, and the resulting concern and anger raises stress levels in the practice area. People who are disorganised, who do not respond to communications from others and do not follow through on tasks tend to cause endless frustration and stress. Other people in the work environment may be overtly stressed, which often has an even greater negative impact. A person who is tense, agitated, monosyllabic and impatient or snaps at colleagues will undoubtedly have a major effect on the work environment. Managing our time and our stress levels is crucial to positive and effective leadership and working relationships. Stress that is badly managed can lead to people feeling harassed and bullied in the working environment.

The difference between being assertive and being aggressive is often not fully understood; a person who thinks that they have just spoken their mind in an assertive manner can have appeared very aggressive to others and alienated them in the process. Knowing how to deal with bullying people and situations can make the difference whether an environment is tolerable or not, but of greater importance is preventing such situations in the first place, as they are so detrimental to staff morale and motivation, and often cause high sickness levels. Thompson (2009) identifies other aspects essential for personal effectiveness (*see* Table 4.1), such as the importance of being creative and realistic, using effective communication and information strategies and making good use of supervision and continuous professional development.

TABLE 4.1 Ten aspects of personal effectiveness (Thompson 2009)

- Self-awareness
- Time management
- Stress management
- Information management
- Assertiveness
- Managing bullying
- Using supervision
- Being creative
- Continuous professional development
- Being realistic

It is clear that Lizzy demonstrated personal effectiveness in her interaction with Zack, and also with the teacher who interrupted the session. She was self-aware and managed her own environment as well as the potential stress caused by the interruption. She was assertive but realistic about other potential interruptions, and she was creative in thinking of ways to solve the problem. We have no knowledge about some of the aspects of personal effectiveness highlighted by Thompson (2009), but her effectiveness was clear in this situation.

One of Lizzy's techniques to manage the situation involved the motivational interviewing approach: she skilfully encouraged Zack to find a solution that he was comfortable with. Motivational interviewing (MI) can be used in any interaction where change is necessary. Primarily, it is used to help the individual to feel empowered to change something in their life, lifestyle or behaviour by using a guiding rather than a directing style. Listening skills are crucial to identify the person's own motivations to change, and to help them identify how this could happen (Rollnick *et al.* 2008). Lizzy used this type of strategy to enable Zack to make choices about how to change the environment he was in so that he felt safer about further interruptions. Lizzy could have taken her own steps to minimise the risk of this happening, which would have reassured her, but would it have reassured Zack? By asking *him* to think of ways that would make him feel safer she let him know that the power stayed with him, and therefore his motivation to stay in the room and carry on talking would have been greater.

Although MI is used in health promotion and behaviour change situations, it is just as applicable in relationships with people in other settings. For example, teams and individuals are often in situations where change needs to take place, but where they face entrenched attitudes that are in line with maintaining the status quo. Rollnick *et al.* (2008) say that people are often perceived as being difficult and non-compliant if they do not want to change. If they are confronted, they will give reasons for things staying the same, and the more they articulate then the more they will want to maintain the status quo. However, nobody is completely unmotivated. We all have our own hopes and aspirations, and by focusing on what we actually want, we can start to see positive ways of achieving it. For example, if Lizzy was to take the situation (of not having uninterrupted private time with students) to the head teacher in a confrontational manner and ask for uninterrupted time, he or she might become defensive. However, if she explored the situation from an MI perspective, she could draw out the head teacher's motivations to provide a suitable environment where students could talk to her about confidential sensitive matters – after all, the drop-in sessions had already been approved for this express purpose. It would be really important to ask the head teacher how to solve the problem, so that they felt more involved in finding a solution, and following it through. This can be a really useful approach to leading change when there are team-dynamic issues, with people becoming more and more entrenched in their views and more resistance to change. This type of team conflict is always counterproductive and generally impacts on the quality of care, and as we discussed in Chapter 2, wastes valuable time and energy.

We often focus on our personal effectiveness as practitioners and ensure that we are fully equipped with all the knowledge and skills to carry out our clinical roles. However, we do not concentrate sufficiently on whether we have developed our *leadership* roles to their maximum effect. This means that we are unable to maximise the service we provide to our patients and clients within the available resources. We need to seize every opportunity to attend any leadership-focused education, whatever our role, so that we can think more broadly and strategically and focus more strongly on solving problems in our practice environments. Such issues could be about our relationships with each other, or our managers, or they could be concerned with better use of time and a better service to our patients and clients. Many people in management positions have had insufficient education and opportunities to develop this expertise, and that can lead to problems. Managers can feel daunted by their roles, pressured on the one hand by practitioners who need them to solve problems or who perhaps are underachieving, and on the other hand by their own managers, who focus exclusively on outcomes. This can lead to managers interfering in situations and disempowering practitioners who are perfectly well able to lead their service forward with minimal intervention. It can also lead to managers being underinvolved with issues of poor performance, and performance management situations being left unaddressed. Neither of these approaches is helpful. In the healthcare environment, we need managers who are genuinely expert in relation to leadership. Such managers can empower people to make clear evidence-based decisions and use resources to best effect, and at the same time support people to develop their clinical and leadership expertise. Morale and motivation will therefore be higher, care will be of a higher standard, and absenteeism, stress, poor performance and burnout will be minimised.

We have discussed how we can actively take a lead in excellent compassionate care by developing positive leadership attributes and developing our personal effectiveness as leaders. Effective change management can make the difference between whether practice development is accepted or not. We will now discuss the potential for effective change management in order to create an environment where excellent compassionate care is the norm.

THOUGHTS FOR YOUR PRACTICE

- Think of examples of situations where you clearly used your high level of self-awareness to good effect. Try to identify situations where you find it harder to be aware of your own impact on situations. How could you develop your self-awareness further?
- What do you struggle with in relation to managing yourself in your professional role? Could your time management be enhanced in any way? Do you think that the level of stress you are experiencing has an impact on your work, and if so, how?
- How could you maximise the way you manage yourself in your work environment? How could you help others to do the same?
- How could you become more assertive in your professional role?
- How could you help others to become more assertive and less aggressive in their work environments?
- Is there any way that you could enhance your personal effectiveness in relation to your leadership? What do you think would help to support you in this?
- How could you use motivational interviewing strategies in your relationships with patients, clients and colleagues? Think of some examples where you could use this approach to maximise the chances of successful outcomes.

KEY THEME TWO – SEEING CHANGE AS A PERSONAL MISSION

ONGOING PRACTICE – DISCUSSION TWO

Lizzy was well aware of the impact of an *actual* interruption, and also of the effect that *potential* breaches in privacy could have, on whether a student felt safe to divulge very sensitive information to her in a school setting. She knew that she needed to try to influence where the drop-in took place and to help members of staff to understand the importance of uninterrupted time where total privacy was respected. She was aware that the teaching staff saw the drop-in as a luxury: somewhere for students to offload minor anxieties in their lives. She knew, however, that these anxieties preyed on their minds, and sometimes involved major disclosures of very traumatic situations. So any attempt to gain the support of teaching staff for the drop-in needed to involve challenging the mindset of the school concerning this service. Lizzy decided that she would approach the head teacher, explain the sensitive issues that could be discussed at these sessions and hopefully get agreement to discuss the matter at the next staff meeting.

She knew that teaching staff would be supportive once they realised the serious nature of the discussions that could take place at the drop-in. This would help her to run a service where privacy was respected, students felt relaxed and comfortable and where the service was as effective as possible.

How can you develop your personal leadership to bring about change?

Lizzy clearly saw taking a lead in developing the school nursing service as a key part of her role. She really was making change happen, and saw change as her personal mission. For change to be effective, practitioners need to understand some of the peripheral issues and relationships that can have an enormous impact on whether change strategies will be effective. Havelock's (1973) theory of change highlights the importance of planning and monitoring the change process. This is best explained using Lizzy as an example, in relation to Havelock's six aspects of change:

➤ Relationship – Lizzy needs to understand the systems within the school and needs to become involved with these systems in order to find ways of initiating the change.

➤ Diagnosis – once she has sufficient understanding of the processes at work, Lizzy has to contemplate ways of increasing awareness of the key issues in order for change to be effective.

➤ Acquire resources for change – Lizzy needs to think about what specific changes need to take place and gather as much information as possible about how these changes could be effected.

➤ Selecting a pathway – Lizzy then thinks about what suggestions she needs to make to maximise her chances of success.

➤ Establish and accept change – Lizzy needs to make sure that changes are accepted and become part of the routine of the school.

➤ Maintenance and separation – once the change has been successful, Lizzy needs to make sure that it is now embedded in the way the drop-ins are perceived within the school. Then she can begin to distance herself, knowing that the change is embedded in the running of the school nursing service.

In order for Havelock's theories to be effective, Lizzy needs to become a change agent and encourage others in her team to be change agents too. It is important to win over the hearts and minds not only of key individuals, but of the organisation as a whole. This is a major challenge, because organisations are notoriously difficult to change. The analogy is often used about how many nautical miles it takes for a large ocean-going vessel to stop moving forwards. The same can be said to be true about changing structures and processes in healthcare, or in this case in education. Effecting change in terms of causing something to happen, or stopping something from happening, takes a strong motivational change agent, a positive mental attitude and a great deal of energy. Change agents need to anticipate resistance and use it to find ways of overcoming problems early, before the problems become too noticeable to those people who might increase the level of resistance to the change process. Understanding the organisation and its cultural norms and processes is essential for success. The change agent has to be an expert communicator to enlist the help of others who understand the issues, and then use their leadership skills to take others with them. Lizzy decided to approach the head teacher first, knowing that he or she would have the power and influence to support any change needed, and would probably also have a strong motivation to enhance the service that the school provided. They also might be supportive of the changes proposed because of their own personality and priorities.

Egan (1994) refers to involved parties as stakeholders, and says that there are nine typical categories of people:

➤ partners – who support your agenda
➤ allies – who will be supportive given encouragement
➤ fellow travellers – who are passive supporters to the agenda but not to you
➤ fence sitters – their allegiance is unclear
➤ loose cannons – may vote against the change just for the sake of it
➤ opponents – they oppose the agenda, but not you personally
➤ adversaries – oppose you and the agenda
➤ bedfellows – support the agenda but may not trust you
➤ voiceless – will be affected but have little power to promote or oppose the change.

There are many reasons why people become resistant to change. We think that it is really important, whenever you need to be effective as a leader, to identify what roles people might take when you are trying to effect change. As we have said, anticipating resistance is important: if we can identify who might be supportive of us, who might be swayed and who will definitely oppose us, we are in a much stronger position to identify strategies that make best use of those who can be most supportive. So being aware of these categories of people can be really helpful when thinking through possible ways of initiating change.

It takes a strong leader with a strong internal locus of control (Rotter 1966), which gives them a sense of having power and influence, to bring about change. It also takes a high degree of self-efficacy (Bandura 1994) for a leader to feel that they can be personally effective in making change happen. These are essential components in taking a lead in developing practice. The likelihood of individuals feeling that they can be successful in bringing about change is greatest if there is a high level of dissatisfaction with the current situation and a low perceived personal risk in relation to leading, or taking part in, the change (Eaton 2010, *see* Figure 4.1).

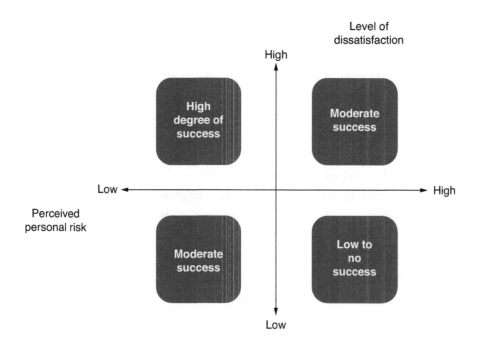

FIGURE 4.1 Personal commitment to change (Eaton 2010)

As a strong advocate for Zack, Lizzy had a high level of dissatisfaction with the drop-in situation because a disturbance could have a high negative impact on a student. She also felt that addressing the problem did not hold a significant personal risk for her because she knew that the school had high standards and would be understanding about the need for privacy, once this was explained.

Her strong self-efficacy and locus of control empowered her to feel able to bring about change.

In some organisations, unfortunately, individuals feel very disempowered and unable to make suggestions or to raise issues in relation to current systems and processes, and this needs to be addressed for any potential change agent to be effective. In an article on the role of the public health midwife, Garrod (2002) highlights five barriers to change, namely:

➤ territorialism – only someone with my job title can do this
➤ traditionalism – we have always done it this way
➤ tribalism – that isn't my role
➤ terrorism – sabotages any change initiatives
➤ timidity – fear of change.

In addition there can be other barriers, for example:

➤ tyranny – you are not allowed to do that
➤ time – we haven't got time to do that.

These are very common reasons why people feel unable to lead or accept change and should be fought on every front, because they are just excuses for not taking changes forward and are based on fear, uncertainty and out-dated norms and values. As Garrod (2002) says, 'If you keep on doing what you have always done, you'll keep on getting what you've always got' (Garrod 2002, p. 532).

In this section, we have discussed how important effective personal leadership is in terms of bringing about change. In the next section, we will go on to discuss how we can effect change, particularly in relation to compassionate care.

THOUGHTS FOR YOUR PRACTICE

● Have you been involved in initiating a change, or been involved with a change led by someone else? If so, how was this change planned and monitored? Have you learnt anything from this experience which you could take forward for future situations?

● How do you think that you could enhance your ability to be a change agent? How could you enhance your communication skills in relation to this?

● How could you plan more in relation to anticipating resistance? How could you use the resistance of others to further develop your thoughts?

- Have you experienced situations where people have taken on stereotypical behaviour in line with Egan's roles, for example, the role of opponent or ally? How could you use this knowledge to help you in the change process?
- Do you feel that you have a strong internal locus of control and high degree of self-efficacy in your work environment? How could you strengthen these further?
- Have you experienced barriers to change in relation to tribalism, territorialism, etc? If so, how could you counter these most effectively in your work situation?

ONGOING PRACTICE – DISCUSSION THREE

Lizzy had the opportunity to discuss with Mark Simpson, the head teacher, how school nursing drop-ins could be more private and confidential. Mark was very understanding about the problems that interruptions could have on sensitive discussions with vulnerable young people. Room availability was problematic within the school, and in other ways the current room was ideal. It was in an area of the school which was busy and where there could be external noise, but generally other students would be unable to see who was going into the room to visit the school nurse. This was seen as an advantage by both Lizzy and Mark, so changing the room did not seem to be the best solution to the problem. The store cupboard in the room was also ideally placed, close to where teaching staff needed to be prior to lessons. It was also one of the few cupboards that could be used to store big items. It seemed that the only solution was for teaching staff to plan ahead the times when they needed to access the cupboard. So the decision was made for Lizzy to attend a staff meeting to explain the problems that interruptions caused in sensitive discussions with students.

At the staff meeting, the problem was raised by the head teacher and Lizzy made sure that in her discussion of the issues, she smiled and made good use of eye contact with all those in the room. She explained that the students were often very embarrassed and reticent to discuss their issues and felt that their problems were minor, when in fact they were very serious. She could see by the looks of concern and nods of the heads that the teaching staff were convinced that this was a real issue. She also clearly acknowledged the difficulties that the teaching staff faced throughout their working day. They started coming up with their own ideas for how to access the cupboard outside the drop-in times. Lizzy left the meeting convinced that the teaching staff understood the issues and would ensure that her sessions were uninterrupted in the future. Therefore, the service she could give to students would be significantly enhanced.

How can you effect change in relation to compassionate care?

Lizzy was clearly successful in her discussions about the drop-in sessions with both the head teacher and other teaching staff at the school. These were sensitive discussions to have, because they involved an organisation in which she was only a visitor. Therefore, tact, diplomacy and advanced communication skills were all needed, as well as a great deal of understanding of the situation from their perspective.

Kotter (1996) discusses an eight-stage model for successful change management. These stages are:

➤ Establish a sense of urgency.
➤ Form a powerful coalition.
➤ Create the right vision.
➤ Communicate the vision.
➤ Empower others.
➤ Plan for and create short-term wins.
➤ Consolidate improvements.
➤ Institutionalise changes.

Establishing a sense of urgency can be difficult when everyone is really busy and there are competing priorities. Often, there is an event that can precipitate the need for a change to be made and is the catalyst for change. Sometimes, however, others need to be convinced that a change is necessary, and evidence might need to be provided from outside the organisation to help to convince them of the need for change. Perceiving the event that has challenged existing practice as an opportunity, and being realistic about strategies that might be successful, are both essential parts of this process.

Forming a powerful coalition, or building a team to take the situation forward, is essential for success. This change team needs to include people with influence, enthusiasm and commitment, and individuals need to see themselves as a team and act as one.

Creating the right vision can be complex because if the vision is not clear, strategies to achieve it will be poorly defined and might prove ineffective.

Communicating the vision involves clear and effective communication of the vision and strategies so that others are engaged and aligned with them, and behaviour is then role-modelled to those who are new to this way of thinking.

Empowering others and empowering action involves removing any obstacles to the change process, and changing procedures and processes that get in the way of the change taking place.

Short-term wins can help people to plan for and achieve visible performance improvements in relation to the change, which should then be acknowledged and rewarded.

Consolidating improvements and *institutionalising change* are essential and involve reinforcing the behaviours that led to the change and helping others to see the connection between new ways of working and a more successful service.

In Lizzy's case, she communicated the urgency of changing the environment in which the drop-ins took place. She included both the head teacher and the teaching staff as members of the change team, and articulated the need for the change. Other members of this team came up with potential solutions, which were much more likely to gain strong acceptance and commitment to the change than if she had suggested them herself, and also helped to dispel any potential negativity towards her or the changes that she was proposing. Once the changes had been agreed, it was important that Lizzy carried on reinforcing the positive behaviour by acknowledging the absence of interruptions and stating how much difference it made to both herself and the young people who attended the drop-ins. It would have been easy not to do this: to simply regard the lack of interruptions as the expected outcome of the change that needed to happen, and feel that no more effort was needed on her part. This would have been a mistake, because planning ahead to avoid interruptions took an effort on the part of the teaching staff; reinforcing the value of the change helped it to become more embedded.

Sometimes it takes this level of intentional effort to create change. An example of this is 'intentional rounding' (Fitzsimons 2011), whereby nurses in hospitals, community hospitals and care homes carry out regular rounds, at set intervals, during which they carry out specific tasks. They are also designed to increase the level of communication and connection with patients in their care. This reduces the randomness of contact, reassures patients that there will be another point of contact soon and encourages nurses to ask patients if there is anything else that they need. This appears to have been successful where it has been adopted – it has been implemented in small ways and then built up to include greater numbers of patients. There was a high emphasis on strong leadership in relation to the implementation and auditing of the change, and it appeared to be important that there was flexibility in relation to how this initiative was introduced. Changes like this can promote a more compassionate environment, because although the rounds are very structured and not initiated on an individual basis, they do ensure that individual contact takes place in a planned manner, which can increase the extent to which patients feel cared about.

As leaders, if we are trying to make changes that raise the standards of care in our practice areas, we need to encourage others to feel positive about themselves and the care that they are providing. This supportive but challenging approach is highlighted by Daloz (1986) in relation to teaching and mentoring. However, the approach is just as important in our relationships with patients, clients and colleagues. If we give high levels of support to somebody, we can also challenge to a high level, because they will feel supported to grow and develop, which will result in a higher level of performance. If, however, we challenge them but do not support them, we are likely to achieve the opposite result – cause them to be demotivated and to draw away from us. If we take the easier option and do not either challenge or support, then we can create a situation, again of low motivation, where there is stasis and apathy. If we are supportive but do not challenge, we reinforce what they are doing or create situations where others simply become role models of ourselves. Neither of

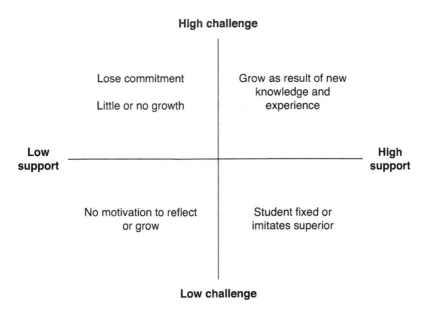

FIGURE 4.2 Effective teaching and mentoring (Daloz 1986)

these approaches leads to development of practice. This is explained graphically in Figure 4.2.

If we want to be leaders who bring about change in relation to compassionate care, we need to create the right balance of challenge and support. We also need to go about change in the most effective ways possible in order to help others see the advantages of specific changes. They will then feel motivated to work alongside us to change aspects of care that need to change, and to develop their own ideas in the process. This will further strengthen us as leaders, and in our leadership role, which in turn will benefit the clients and patients in our care.

THOUGHTS FOR YOUR PRACTICE

- What change would you like to make in practice? Use Kotter's eight-stage model (1996) to plan this change. How will this positively impact on patients or clients in your care?
- Think of a recent change that has been implemented in your practice area. Were efforts made to reinforce and consolidate this change? If not, was this change maintained? What have you learnt specifically that would be helpful in terms of making change part of the normal way of doing things in your practice area?
- Are there any examples of ways in which you could build in intentional processes to improve care in your area? If so, what would you like to implement as intentional and planned interventions? How would you achieve this?
- What could you do to increase the amount of challenge and support within your team in relation to patient care? Develop workable strategies to build these into your usual practice role.

SUMMARY

Throughout this chapter, we have discussed the essential role a positive attitude is in relation to delivering excellent and compassionate nursing care. We have emphasised the role of strong leadership in relation to making this standard of care the norm, and in challenging standards of care that we are not happy with.

So how do we personally take the lead in creating this environment, and what attributes do we need to demonstrate in order to be effective? We need to look at what our patients and clients are saying, and what they are not saying. These hidden messages can hold the key to enhanced care. This applies to our colleagues, too. They might have excellent ideas that would help us to deliver better and more individualised care which do not involve more resources. We need to be resonant leaders who demonstrate high levels of emotional intelligence and emotional brilliance. We have seen too many examples of dissonant leaders who are far removed from the mindset and priorities of staff who are caring for patients. Some of them are frankly alexithymic, emotionally tone-deaf and do not understand the feelings of those they manage, their colleagues or their patients or clients. Some people develop that sort of attitude in their work environment to protect themselves against the pressures of their work, but the attitude is very counterproductive to leading practice forward in a positive way. Our own personality can have a strong impact on our team morale and motivation. If we do not demonstrate a high level of self-awareness and do not have positive self-regard, then we are likely not to have sufficient self-control to manage our behaviour and act as positive role models to others in our team, Students, new team members and people in our care will find it difficult to know how to react to us if we are unpredictable and do not demonstrate control over our emotions. We need to use all of our emotional intelligence and other intelligences to bring out the best in ourselves and others.

To be personally effective as leaders, we need to be able to manage ourselves and understand what makes us personally effective in our roles as practitioners and as leaders. We need to use such strategies as assertiveness, good time management and motivational interviewing to bring about positive change where we can.

We need to see change as a personal mission so that change can be seen as something that is positive and ongoing, rather than challenging and difficult. We need to plan for change, expect resistance and use this in a positive way, and then monitor changes that have been introduced. This needs us to be change agents, who have excellent communication skills, have a clear understanding of what it takes to be personally effective, understand what barriers to change there could be and have an internal locus of control. We need to know who our allies are and who our adversaries could be, and use clear strategies that will increase our effectiveness in adversarial situations where change is seen only as a challenge, to be stopped at all costs.

When we are effective in our change strategies, we will develop systems that will enhance patient care. We will implement intentional and proactive ways forward, as well as more reactive and individual problem-solving approaches.

We will monitor these changes and ensure that these new strategies are embedded into our culture. We will also plan for change in structured ways and use our excellent communication skills to support and challenge ourselves and those in our team to strive to deliver ever better care.

A report which analysed a sample of critical patient comments was posted on the UK Patient Opinion website in 2011, and staff attitude was perceived as crucial to good care (www.patientopinion.org.uk). Thirty-three per cent of postings raised staff attitudes as being a concern, with insufficient care and compassion highlighted by 30% of patients. Poor communication, lack of responsiveness, choice of providers, dignity and inclusivity were also raised as concerns. However, it is important to point out that 79% of the responses expressed positive views about their experiences of healthcare. In these positive reports, staff attitudes were also perceived as the most common aspect of the very best care experienced by patients and their carers. Quality of care was not measured just by the quality of the medical outcomes. This clearly demonstrates how important it is to patients to be nursed by people with positive nurse attitudes. We need to take a lead in ensuring that this is the case.

REFERENCES

Ashburner C, Meyer J, Johnson B, *et al.* Using action research to address loss of personhood in a continuing care setting. *Illn Crises Loss.* 2004; **12**(1): 23–37.

Bandura A. Self-efficacy. In: Ramachandran VS, editor. *Encyclopedia of Human Behaviour.* Volume 4. New York: Academic Press; 1994. pp. 71–81.

Cassidy T. *Stress, Cognition and Health.* London: Routledge; 1999.

Chambers C, Ryder E. *Compassion and Caring in Nursing.* Oxford: Radcliffe Publishing; 2009.

Chapman M. *Emotional Intelligence Pocketbook.* Alresford: Management Pocketbooks; 2001.

Cummings G, Hayduk L, Estabrooks C. Mitigating the impact of hospital restructuring on nurses. *Nurs Res.* 2005; **54**(1): 2–12.

Daloz L. *Effective Teaching and Mentoring: realizing the transformational power of adult learning experiences.* San Francisco, CA: Jossey-Bass; 1986.

Earley P, Ang S. Cultural intelligence: individual interactions across cultures. 2003. In: Berry J, Poortinga Y, Breugelmans S, *et al. Cross-Cultural Psychology: research and application.* Cambridge: Cambridge University Press; 2011.

Eaton M. Why change programmes fail. *Training J.* 2010 Feb; 53–7. Available at: www.trainingjournal.com/feature/2010-02-01-why-change-programmes-fail (accessed 11 December 2011).

Egan G. Working the shadow side: a guide to positive behind-the-scenes management. 1994. In: Buchanan D, Huczynski A. *Organisational Behaviour: an introductory text.* 8th ed. London: Prentice Hall; 2004.

Fitzsimons B, Bartley A, Cornwell J. Intentional rounding: its role in supporting essential care. *Nurs Times*. 2011; **107**(27): 18–21.

Furnham A. *Management Intelligence: sense and nonsense for the successful manager.* Hampshire: Palgrave Macmillan; 2008.

Garrod D. Sure start: the role of the public health midwife. *MIDIRS Midwif Dig*. 2002; **12**(Suppl. 1): S32–5.

Goleman D. *Emotional Intelligence: why it can matter more than IQ.* London: Bloomsbury Publishing; 1996.

Goleman D, Boyatzis R, McKee A. Appendix B: Emotional intelligence leadership competencies. In: Goleman D, Boyatzis R, McKee A. *The New Leaders: transforming the art of leadership into the science of results.* London; Sphere; 2002.

Gudykunst W, Hammer M. Basic training design: approaches in intercultural training. 1983. In: Berry J, Poortinga Y, Breugelmans S, *et al. Cross-Cultural Psychology: research and application.* Cambridge: Cambridge University Press; 2011.

Havelock R. *The Change Agent's Guide to Innovation in Education.* Englewood Cliffs, NJ: Educational Technology; 1973.

Hein S. *EQ for Everybody: a practical guide to emotional intelligence.* Clearwater, FL: Aristotle Press; 1996.

Horton-Deutsch S, Sherwood G. Reflection: an educational strategy to develop emotionally competent nurse leaders. *J Nurs Manag*. 2008; **16**(8): 946–54.

Jopson N. The ice cream that changed my approach to nursing. *Nurs Times*. 2010; **106**(20): 10.

Kotter J. *Leading Change.* USA: Harvard Business Press; 1996.

Newton V. Teach students compassion by being an excellent role model. *Nurs Times*. 2010; **106**(39): 10.

Nicholson C, Flatley M, Wilkinson C, *et al.* Everybody matters 1: how getting to know your patients helps to promote dignified care. *Nurs Times*. 2010a; **106**(20): 12–14.

Nicholson C, Flatley M, Wilkinson C, *et al.* Everybody matters 2: promoting dignity in acute care through effective communication. *Nurs Times*. 2010b; **106**(21): 12–14.

Nicholson C, Flatley M, Wilkinson C. Everybody matters 3: engaging patients and relatives in decision making to promote dignity. *Nurs Times*. 2010c; **106**(22): 10–12.

Peterson C, Seligman M. *Character Strengths and Virtues: a handbook and classification.* Oxford: Oxford University Press; 2004.

Radcliffe M. Do you have the emotional intelligence of a Muppet? *Nurs Times*. 2010; **106**(3): 25.

Rollnick S, Miller W, Butler C. *Motivational Interviewing in Health Care: helping patients change behavior.* London: Guilford Press; 2008.

Rotter J. Generalised expectancies for internal versus external control of reinforcement. *Psychol Monogr*. 1966; **80**: 1–28.

Rowan K. *Grumpy Nurse Did Not Tell Me Her Name, Smile at Me or Calm Me.* 2009. Available at: www.nursingtimes.net/whats-new-in-nursing/students/student-blog-archive/grumpy-nurse-did-not-tell-me-her-name-smile-at-me-or-calm-me/50007204.blog (accessed 11 December 2011).

Rungapadiachy D. *Interpersonal Communication and Psychology for Healthcare Professionals.* Oxford: Butterworth Heinemann; 1999.

Rungapadiachy D. *Self Awareness in Health Care: engaging in helping relationships.* Hampshire: Palgrave Macmillan; 2008.

Santry C. We need to be clear about our primary responsibility. *Nurs Times.* 2010; **106**(4): 4–5.

Santry C. Patient communication still weak. *Nurs Times.* 2010; **106**(20): 5.

Schon D. *Educating the Reflective Practitioner: toward a new design for teaching and learning in the professions.* San Francisco, CA: Jossey-Bass; 1987.

Seligman M. *Helplessness: On depression, development and death.* San Francisco, CA: WH Freeman; 1975.

Sifneos P. Affect, emotional conflict and deficit: an overview. Psychotherapy-and-psychosomatics. 1972. In: Goleman D. *Emotional Intelligence: why it can matter more than IQ.* London: Bloomsbury Publishing; 1996.

Thompson N. *People Skills.* 3rd ed. Basingstoke: Palgrave Macmillan; 2009.

www.NHSLeadershipQualities.nhs.uk (2006) and revised www.nhsleadership.org.uk/framework.asp (2011).

www.patientopinion.org.uk/resources/POreport2011.pdf

Conclusion: Excellence in compassionate nursing care – how will you take the lead?

Overview of the chapter

Key theme one – why is compassion central to excellent nursing care?

- Case study 5.1
- How does compassionate care stay central to your nursing practice?
- Thoughts for your practice
- Ongoing practice – discussion one
- What are the potential challenges to enhancing compassionate care?
- Thoughts for your practice

Key theme two – how can you take the lead on enhancing a compassionate culture within your practice environment?

- Ongoing practice – discussion two
- What positive leadership principles will you use to ensure that excellence is central to nursing care?
- Thoughts for your practice
- Ongoing practice – discussion three
- How will you take the lead in making sure that change is ongoing in pursuit of excellent nursing care?
- Thoughts for your practice

Summary

References

OVERVIEW OF THE CHAPTER

In the previous chapters, we have highlighted how crucial nurses are in relation to leading practice forward and in creating a positive culture in their practice environment. Today's resource-stretched healthcare environment is undoubtedly stressful for all health and social care practitioners, and it can seem as if individuals are powerless to make changes they believe are needed. Patient and client needs are greater than ever, and the vulnerability they feel is potentially very disempowering. We need to speak up for those who cannot or do not feel confident to speak for themselves, or who feel lost in an organisation that seems frightening, uncaring and disempowering. If we as nurses do not speak up and make a difference, then who will?

However, we can also feel as if we do not have a voice in today's healthcare environment. Our pleas for higher staffing levels are ignored, safety issues can go unaddressed and all that seems to matter are targets and outcomes set by people who do not seem to understand the stressors that we deal with on a daily basis.

This is why we need to use our leadership knowledge and skills to their greatest effect. Many trusts are investing in leadership study days and courses to try to increase the level of leadership throughout their healthcare environments, so it is important to seize these opportunities whenever they become available.

We need to consider alternative ways of taking a lead in excellent and compassionate care. We need to analyse potential barriers to achieving this high level of care, such as inadequate resourcing, the culture of our practice areas and our own individual attitudes (Chambers and Ryder 2009). When practice in our wards and clinical environments falls short of absolute excellence, whether regularly or only occasionally, it is our role to make a difference. Small differences can mean everything to someone in our care, and small differences can be the beginnings of even greater differences that overcome the barriers hindering our quality of care.

In summing up, excellence in compassionate nursing care is the key to nursing practice, and leadership is key to making this happen. Practitioners need to be valued and empowered in order to make this vital difference to a patient's or client's experience of care, and leadership is everybody's responsibility. This multidimensional, multicultural and multifaceted environment in which we work is highly complex. Responses to change are required very fast, and effective leadership skills are essential to keep excellence in compassionate care at the forefront of practice.

We would like you to ask yourself four critical questions:

➤ What are the barriers to excellent practice in our practice areas, and what are the potential ways forward?

➤ How can we continue to take a lead on excellent care in the resource-driven environment of health and social care today?

➤ How do we influence the practice culture of where we work so that excellence remains central to practice?

➤ How can we use our own personal values, beliefs and attributes to take a lead on excellent and compassionate practice?

As mentioned in Chapter 1, Goodrich (2009) highlights the connection between relational and transactional aspects of care. She says that when both are present, then care is as it should be and everything works (*see* Figure 5.1). However, when the structures are in place but relationships are lacking, things feel efficient but impersonal, and where structures are lacking but relationships are strong, practice can feel caring but chaotic. If both structures and relationships are lacking, this is the worst of both worlds and things feel unpleasant and inefficient. If our practice areas feel like this to us, we can be sure that people in our care feel it to an even greater extent. After all, they do not have the freedom to leave at the end of a shift, and they have very little ability to change their circumstances for the better.

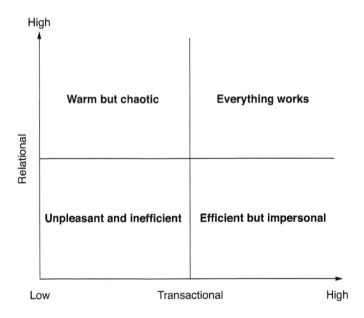

FIGURE 5.1 Transactional and relational aspects of care (Goodrich 2009)

In this closing chapter, we ask two key questions: why is compassion central to excellent nursing care, and how can you take the lead on enhancing a compassionate culture within your practice environment? We hope that by discussing these questions, we can help you to create action plans with achievable and measurable goals to ensure that you do take that lead and that practice benefits as a result.

KEY THEME ONE – WHY IS COMPASSION CENTRAL TO EXCELLENT NURSING CARE?

CASE STUDY 5.1

Jim had never been a patient in hospital, and he did not want to be admitted to one now. He had visited his wife, Ellen, there when she was seriously ill, and it had frightened him. The nurses were very caring of her, he had felt reassured by the way they talked to her and seemed to genuinely care about what was important to her. However, some days when he visited, Ellen would be lying in bed without her dentures and without her hair brushed; she would have hated to be seen like that because she always took such pride in her appearance. She looked frankly scared and disorientated. There had been too many days like that before she died, and he realised how vulnerable everyone was when they were ill or were recovering from surgery.

But he also knew that he really could not manage any longer without a hip replacement. The pain was severe, mobility of any kind was becoming a problem and he was becoming unable to care for himself. Jim gritted his teeth and approached the preadmission clinic reception. The receptionist immediately looked up and smiled at him, and it was clear that she knew who he was and why he was there as soon as he said his name. She told a nurse who had just approached the reception area that he had arrived. The nurse introduced herself as Jasmine and said that she had just one more thing to do and would be with him in a couple of minutes. He had heard that said to his wife before and she would still be waiting an hour later, so he was pleasantly surprised when, true to her word, she came over to him a few minutes later. She asked him if he had been to this hospital before, and to his immense embarrassment he felt tears well up in his eyes when he said that his wife had died there 8 months ago. She immediately put her hand on his arm and took him to a private area. She could see that he was embarrassed, but she also seemed to know how scared he was. She asked if there was anything she could do to help him to feel better about being back in the hospital where he had been through so much in the past. He was surprised to find that he was actually feeling much better just by knowing that Jasmine understood how he felt. He hoped that the other nurses would be as sensitive as she was.

How does compassionate care stay central to your nursing practice?

As we discussed previously, nurses in today's healthcare environment often feel:

➤ disillusioned
➤ disempowered
➤ angry
➤ stressed
➤ unappreciated
➤ burnt out
➤ undervalued
➤ tired
➤ criticised
➤ under fire
➤ defensive.

Additionally, they may feel:

➤ anxious about a patient or client
➤ concerned about further deterioration
➤ unsupported by their managers
➤ worried about lack of supervision opportunities
➤ in need of greater skills in relation to aspects of care
➤ on a hamster wheel going faster and faster
➤ unable to raise issues and put their head above the parapet
➤ unable to mobilise resources or think strategically
➤ unable to make a difference.

This is understandable, because the media tend to operate in an environment of deficit journalism that generates a barrage of articles about care that has fallen short of standards, and rarely if ever report on excellent care. There is talk of 'always' and 'never' events, and yet 'never' events still seem to happen and 'always' events are far from the norm, and that is very demoralising. Nurses, if asked, would say that they should 'always' respect those in their care and listen to their views about what is important to them. They would also say that patients should 'never' feel disempowered, frightened and uncared for. Unfortunately, this is often not the case. In the UK, the Healthcare Commission's damning report into failings in the Mid Staffordshire Foundation Trust (Francis 2010) highlighted that minimum standards were not being met. The chair of the trust, Sir Stephen Moss, commented that nurses had the technological expertise to care for patients, but did not necessarily recognise the importance of doing so with care and compassion. He said that nurses should stop defending their profession when poor care has been highlighted, and should accept responsibility for improving standards of care.

Although the comments are bound to alienate and anger some nurses, others would acknowledge that there is some truth in them, and that despite resource constraints, compassion should move higher up the list of nursing priorities and not be seen as an add-on.

Jasmine was undoubtedly under a lot of pressure when Jim came to see her that morning. However, she did not lose sight of his individual needs and used her considerable communication skills to reassure him and gain insight into his feelings, despite her work pressures. She did not need to spend much time doing this, but it had an immense impact on him and his anxiety. This would probably have saved valuable time later in his hospital stay and was an excellent use of her time and skills. Sometimes we need to look for ways in which to reduce patient and client stress levels at an early point in our contact with them. Otherwise we, or our colleagues, end up spending much more time in giving greater reassurance, dealing with angry outbursts or upset patients, or perhaps dealing with complaints. So not only should Jasmine's level of compassion be central to any nurse's practice – it is also an excellent use of resources.

Some cultures view compassion as key to their way of life; for example, the Hawaiian aloha spirit is built into Hawaiian law and is tangible to people who visit and live in the Hawaiian Islands. The aloha spirit involves kindness, tenderness, unity, pleasantness, humility and perseverance, and these are what should be reflected in compassionate nursing care. Dr Norman Estin, who works for Doctors On Call in western Maui says, 'At our Doctors On Call medical offices, we specifically try to greet each visitor and patient with a mindful "Aloha" and do the same when they are leaving. The word conveys the spirit of a warm, friendly, caring welcome or departure as well as usually bringing a pause and a smile. It also helps us to avoid using inappropriate or counterproductive comments, like "Did you want to see Doctor?" or "Hope you feel better!"' (Estin, in Ellman and Santos 2010, p. 192).

It is interesting how small touches like this really do matter, how they reduce stress in patients and clients, and increase morale and motivation in staff and make them feel more supported in their roles. We are more likely to be thanked for carrying out care, which in turn helps us to feel valued and appreciated. Max Pemberton, who is himself a doctor, was admitted following an acute medical emergency and says that it was the 'tiny, insignificant things that made all the difference. A kind word, a thoughtful gesture, a sympathetic smile: these are the things that there are no tick boxes for, and that are so difficult to regulate or control; yet for the patient, are so important' (Pemberton 2010). Jasmine clearly understood the importance of these small touches in her contact with Jim, and as a result his stress levels decreased enormously.

Jason Leitch, national lead for quality in the Scottish government, spoke at the second international conference on compassionate care in Edinburgh in 2011, and he made two points that particularly resonated with us. First, he talked about his grandmother's emergency admission to the accident and emergency department following a major stroke. He said that because people were aware of his role and status, they were making special efforts to ensure that quality care was being provided. However, the doctor, who stayed on duty over and above his working hours (which was sensitive and caring), did not wash his hands before carrying out an intervention involving his grandmother. Leitch made the point that by failing to say anything at that moment, he himself changed from being an articulate patient advocate to being a disempowered grandson who could not speak up to protect his grandmother from potential infection issues. He said that if that could happen to him, how much more likely was it to happen to someone with less personal and professional confidence?

Leitch's second point was about 'Lauren's list'. This was an initiative that was developed after Lauren, an adolescent girl having chemotherapy, complained about the care that she was receiving. The chief executive of the trust came to visit her and asked her what she felt was lacking and what could be done to improve her care. She did not ask for the leukaemia to go away or for the chemo to stop, but just asked for the following: for people to say who they were and what their role was when they approached her to say what they were going to do; to tell her if they were going to touch her and tell her if it was going to hurt; and to say goodbye when they were leaving. That was not asking a great deal and should have been happening anyway, so her requests were written on a board outside her room and called 'Lauren's list'. This approach was adopted for other patients on the ward, who also had their own lists of things that were important to them. Other practice areas have used this approach to ask patients' relatives and carers to communicate what they would like to happen in relation to their loved one's care that day. Other practice areas use 'get to know you boards' to invite patients to say what their hobbies and achievements are, what they like to be called, what stresses them and what makes them happy.

Garrison Keillor, the well-known American author, commented on how the little things really matter from a patient's perspective. He says that 'Nurses are smart and brisk and utterly capable. They bring some humour to the situation. ("Care for some jewellery?" she says as she puts the wristband on me.) . . . The women who draw blood samples at Mayo do it gently with a whole litany of small talk to ease the little blip of puncture, and "Here it comes" and the needle goes in, and "Sorry about that," and I feel some human tenderness there, as if she thought, "I could be the last woman to hold that dude's hand." A brief sweet moment of common humanity' (Keillor 2009). These clear demonstrations of humanity are so meaningful for patients, clients and their families, and it is all too easy to underestimate their value and importance.

Ruth Bailey, who is herself a practice nurse in the UK, talks very movingly about her experiences when her father became acutely and critically unwell following a massive haemorrhage after routine surgery. She says that 'I have always known that it is the little things that make a difference but to really feel this is something else. Little things, said and done, have the power to make the situation bearable or to amplify distress' (Bailey 2011, p. 11). She gives examples of how all members of staff had the power to make this difference, from a healthcare assistant who brought her coffee in the middle of the night, to the staff nurse who sat with her in supportive silence when she was waiting to hear if her father had survived, to the ward clerk who looked after her overnight bags and to all those who tried to satisfy the family's constant need for information. However, she also experienced insensitivity, for example, when a ward sister criticised her for using the wrong exit on an unfamiliar ward; a lack of understanding of her concern when her father's feed had been delayed for 12 hours; and a staff nurse who told her not to worry while he was suctioning 300 mL of blood from her father's tube. As she says, 'I know as well as the next nurse that sometimes you have to wait. Now I know the agony waiting brings'. She goes on to say that:

It was the high-tech, high-intervention stuff that saved my dad, but it was the attention to detail that truly made the difference. I found enormous comfort in the way the nurses supported his swollen sausage fingers on little rolled-up towels, and wrote his favourite programmes on the whiteboard near his bed. When they remembered not to speak into his deaf ear, I knew he mattered. I was touched when they remembered my name and told him I was there . . . Thoughtless care and shoddy nursing, while upsetting, were outweighed by compassion. Yet shoddy care exists and is tolerated. It needs to be named and rectified for not only the distress it causes but also the dilution of care and the damage it does to the profession. Small acts of caring kept the family going. We need to treasure this ability and foster its growth. It is easy to underestimate the impact of nursing actions. When you are in the middle of a maelstrom, good nursing is everything. (Bailey 2011, p. 11)

The NHS ombudsman's report into NHS care of older people (Abraham 2011, p. 8) says that 'The NHS touches our lives at times of basic human need when care and compassion are what matter most.' It is very important that all nurses remember this important point. After all, we and our loved ones are potential recipients of care, and the vulnerability and the centrality of compassion at that crucial time should be key to everything we do. It might just be a moment in the day for us as nurses, but how we communicate might be something that is remembered for the rest of someone's life.

We do need to recognise that these are all really important aspects of the art of nursing and must not get so wrapped up with the science and technology of our roles that we fail to practise the art of what we do best. We need to be effective role models of the art of nursing and help our more junior, and senior, colleagues to also act as positive role models, and so inspire others still further. Armstrong (2011) highlights the importance of showing compassion for ourselves, as well as others, and yet healthcare environments are often some of the least compassionate environments to work in. If this is the case, how can we show compassion to others when we are not treated with compassion by colleagues and more senior managers? A more compassionate practice culture is essential for patients and staff alike.

THOUGHTS FOR YOUR PRACTICE

- What would be 'always' and 'never' events in your practice environment? If you find these have focused on preventing emergencies in care, now try to apply them to communication strategies and best care.
- How can you work harder at delivering technological expertise with care and compassion? How would you be the most effective role model to others?
- How can you make compassion absolutely central to all patient or client care, and not merely an add-on?
- What could you do to reduce patient or client stress at an early point in your contact with them?
- Do you think that you could develop your own 'aloha spirit' in your practice environment? If so, how?
- Think about what small touches would be important to you if you were a patient or client in your practice environment. What small differences could you make to enhance the care that you give? How could you share these thoughts with others in your team?
- How could you empower patients and their loved ones to feel more able to express what is important to them?
- Could you see a way of introducing 'Lauren's list'-type strategies in your practice area? If so, how?
- How could you work towards creating a more caring environment for your colleagues? How could you be a more effective role model for others?

ONGOING PRACTICE – DISCUSSION ONE

Jasmine arrived at work feeling rather tired and dispirited. The bus had been late, and she had had to walk much more briskly than usual to get there on time. As it was pouring with rain, that would probably have been necessary anyway, but it was not the best start to the day. The rest of the preadmission team seemed equally demoralised. She made herself a quick cup of coffee, and then saw an envelope with her name on it. That was unusual. Usually any communications were from senior managers about things that would give them all extra things to do, but the writing on the envelope gave the impression of a personal letter.

When Jasmine opened the letter, she was taken aback to see that it was from Jim. She had to think hard to remember who Jim was as she saw so many patients every day. However, she remembered how frightened he had seemed and how she had tried to reassure him. Jim's words were very humbling because they said how important her sensitive approach had been and how he had then felt able to agree to the operation that had benefited him so much. She felt that she had only done what any nurse would do, but clearly from reading Jim's letter she could see that in his experience that had not been the case. She started to think about ways of ensuring that they used a sensitive approach with all patients who seemed unusually nervous and concerned. She decided to discuss this with her colleagues. After all, if her attitude had made so much difference to Jim, this would be important for others coming to the preadmission clinic too.

What are the potential challenges to enhancing compassionate care?

Jim clearly felt as if he had been treated as an individual and in a genuinely caring manner by Jasmine, so much so that he took the time to express his gratitude in writing. However, Jasmine was exceptionally busy in her nursing role, and if asked, she would have said she felt as if she never had enough time to give to each of the patients who came to her clinic.

Throughout this book, we have discussed the potential challenges to excellent and compassionate care, namely resource constraints, culture of the practice environment and individual nurse attitude. In our first book, we identified several potential challenges to compassionate care that could be resource based, for example:

➤ time constraints
➤ inadequate staffing levels
➤ fragmentation of care
➤ limited time to build relationships
➤ focus on outcomes and targets
➤ increased technology
➤ 'too busy to care'.

Jasmine clearly was restricted in the time she had to give to individual patients and had limited time to build relationships. There were probably occasions when there was inadequate staffing, and like every nursing area, there would have been numerous targets to meet. The emphasis would have been on ensuring that every patient was fit for their planned surgery and that all relevant tests had been carried out to ensure that this was the case. However, this did not prevent Jasmine from being able to identify emotional distress in one of her patients, for example Jim, nor prevent her from being able to show her humanity and nursing expertise by reassuring him and demonstrating that she genuinely cared.

In relation to the culture of a practice area, we identified other challenges to excellent nursing care (Chambers and Ryder 2009), for example:

➤ stereotyping people and acceptance of non-inclusive and judgemental attitudes
➤ cultural norms and values being misunderstood
➤ culture of the environment not promoting sensitive care
➤ lack of leadership focusing on compassionate care
➤ inappropriately high focus on outcomes and task centred.

Jasmine was possibly working in an area where the individual needs of patients *were* seen as a priority. However, she could have been working in an area which did not support or encourage sensitive care and where there was a lack of understanding of individual patient needs, with no leadership to encourage this approach. The focus could have been on how many patients were seen rather than on whether their needs had been met at the end of their appointment.

Individual nurse attitude we saw as being key to overcoming the pressures of care that make patients and clients feel undervalued and not cared for, and we identified challenges here too (Chambers and Ryder 2009), for example, when nurses demonstrated the following attitudes or behaviours:

➤ stress and anxiety
➤ being judgemental
➤ insensitive care
➤ emotional overload
➤ distancing themselves from the patient in their care
➤ poor sense of humour
➤ personal moral or emotional distress
➤ lack of empathy
➤ overemphasis on the science of nursing and insufficient emphasis in the art of nursing.

Jasmine did not show any sign of these tendencies; maybe she was able to overcome any potentially negative feelings when she was in a one-to-one relationship with patients and therefore could act with compassion, as she did with Jim. She was clearly empathetic, consistent with Middleton's observation (2011) that nurses do not have to experience every situation that their patients or clients do in order to see things from their perspective.

As nurses, we need to challenge unsafe resources and a prevailing culture in our practice areas which allows insensitive care to continue. We need to take a lead and be positive role models by ensuring that we behave with sensitivity and compassion, and encourage our colleagues to do the same. We need to be mentors to our students and help them to understand the importance of being sensitive and non-judgemental at all times. We cannot rely on these attitudinal skills to be taught in the university curriculum, and we have a responsibility to teach and emulate them in our practice curriculum too. Case studies and patient perspectives should be used as much as possible to help students develop these skills. We need to challenge substandard, unkind or insensitive care and not just carry on going faster and faster on the hamster wheel trying to do more and more to meet ever-increasing targets. Inappropriate cultural and attitudinal issues need to be challenged by all of us, and we should encourage our students and junior team members to be our harshest critics. This is the only way to meet the challenges of ensuring excellent and compassionate care in our practice areas.

THOUGHTS FOR YOUR PRACTICE

- In what ways could you enhance the focus on building relationships and identifying emotional distress in patients and clients, despite your busy working environment and your very real time constraints? How could you take a lead in encouraging others to do the same?
- Try to identify particular ways in which individual patient and client needs could have higher priority in your practice environment. How could you influence the culture of the environment to ensure that the quality of the patient's experience is perceived as just as important as quantitative outcome measures?
- You cannot have experienced every aspect of your patients' or clients' situations, but how could you enhance your understanding of how situations and care could feel from their perspectives? How could you use this as a learning tool for others in your team?
- What situations would make you take a stand and challenge systems or substandard practice? Do you need to rethink the point at which you might try to make that vital difference? How could you work with colleagues to do the same?

KEY THEME TWO – HOW CAN YOU TAKE THE LEAD ON ENHANCING A COMPASSIONATE CULTURE WITHIN YOUR PRACTICE ENVIRONMENT?

ONGOING PRACTICE – DISCUSSION TWO

Jasmine waited for the right opportunity to raise the subject of Jim's feedback with her colleagues. She felt a bit wary of bringing it up because she had only recently qualified and had not been working in the clinic long, whereas her colleagues had been working there for some time. One day, when the preadmission clinic was quiet, the timing seemed right. She commented to her two nursing colleagues, Jo and Francis, that although she had always focused on what questions needed to be asked and what tests needed to be carried out when patients attended the clinic, she had never really considered how stressed they might be about their imminent admission. She then described how her experience with Jim had made her aware of how past healthcare experiences could either be reassuring to patients or could make them feel more anxious, and how this awareness seemed to be helping her to build a relationship with them in the short time she had available.

Jasmine explained that she had now started to ask how they felt about their upcoming admission. She was surprised that it did not seem to take her any longer to carry out the assessments, and patients seemed to be more relaxed and smiled as they left the room. She also had positive feedback from colleagues on the wards that patients seemed more relaxed on admission. They seemed to know what to expect, had fewer questions and generally seemed to require less time from staff in terms of needing reassurance. From Jasmine's point of view, the appointments seemed to go more smoothly, she felt much more positive about her role in the admissions process and felt that she was genuinely getting to know patients individually. The clinic was running to time, despite her asking them extra questions about how they were feeling and what information they would find helpful, which was also an improvement. She thought this was because she was no longer giving routine information to all patients, some of which was not needed, but was concentrating instead on answering their specific questions.

Jasmine was surprised that, considering their seniority, Jo and Francis seemed really interested in how she asked questions and how she had found that this approach worked best. She described various situations when she felt that it had helped during an appointment. They seemed genuinely interested and wanted to talk about it again after trying it themselves. Jasmine left at the end of the day feeling valued, and feeling that she had contributed something to the service that would help patients to receive a more tailored approach based on their specific requirements, needs and anxieties.

What positive leadership principles will you use to ensure that excellence is central to nursing care?

Jasmine clearly demonstrated her leadership in this situation. She was aware of the resource issues and the time constraints that her service struggled with. However, she took an individualistic approach to practice herself, and took a lead on influencing the practice of others and trying to influence the prevailing target-driven culture in which she worked.

Resourcing, the challenge we discussed in Chapter 2, is always going to be an issue in today's healthcare environment, but Jasmine used certain principles to bring positive approaches into her day-to-day practice. We believe the following positive principles are essential when struggling with resource limitations:

➤ Challenge inadequate resources when they affect care.
➤ Understand that service can always benefit from more resources.
➤ Maximise the use of current resources.
➤ Focus on the quality and not just quantity of care.
➤ Focus on what patients and clients value.
➤ Try to maintain continuity of care whenever possible.
➤ Make the most effective use of the skills of different members of the team.
➤ Keep motivation alive.

The second challenge, focused on in Chapter 3, is that of the culture of the environment. We believe that applying the following positive principles will improve the culture of our practice environments:

➤ Take a lead in promoting a positive practice culture.
➤ Challenge poor care in a supportive and educational manner.
➤ Create a positive team environment and good team dynamics.
➤ Encourage feedback from patients and clients.
➤ Work in partnership with those in our care.
➤ Focus on enhancing care.
➤ Make change a personal mission.

The third and final challenge for us, which formed the focus of Chapter 4, is that of individual nurse attitude. The positive principles for improving our own attitudes to practice are as follows:

➤ Review communication skills.
➤ Support colleagues who are finding it difficult to cope.
➤ Challenge insensitive care and judgemental attitudes.
➤ Seek feedback on behaviours and standards in practice.
➤ Do not pass on nurse stress to people we provide a service for.
➤ Focus on the individual and building up a therapeutic relationship, however brief.
➤ Ensure that an ethos of positive practice is embedded in the practice environment.

We know that these principles are not easy to maintain in the highly stressed and sometimes demoralised environments where we work, but if we do, we enhance patient and client care, reduce complaints, enhance morale and motivation and reduce sickness and absence levels.

Hodgetts (2011) says good leaders can be recognised when you see them, but it is difficult to define what good leadership is. She says that the five essential characteristics of a good leader are:

➤ constancy aligned with trust and being genuine
➤ being able to make healthy relationships within the working environment
➤ staying focused and consistent
➤ thinking of the organisation rather than your own position
➤ creating a culture of healthy living and healthy working (Hodgetts 2011).

Rafferty (2011) adds to the 'good leadership' discussion by suggesting that leaders should lead by example, using Florence Nightingale as the epitome of a nurse who believed in compassion and saw how small touches mattered. She says that challenges in care are not new, but we need to recognise the fact that organisations sometimes fail the most vulnerable people in our society. If we acknowledge that there is a problem and take responsibility for working out why the problem exists, we can understand why we sometimes fall short of the standards we would like to achieve. As Rafferty (2011) says, 'Clarity of purpose, moral courage and a coalition for action was Nightingale's response to the call. We need to do likewise – to light and lead the way' (p. 11).

As Adams (2010) and the King's Fund report (2011) say, leadership should be part of everyone's role, at whatever level you work. This can mean having the confidence to speak out for others, which takes courage. Prescott (2010) says, 'True leadership is not about having the benefit of hindsight. It is about having the gift of vision, courage and compassion'.

THOUGHTS FOR YOUR PRACTICE

- How do you think that you could use your own personal motivation to enhance care in your practice area?
- In what ways could you maximise your resources so patients or clients receive the best care possible within the constraints that you have?
- How could you influence the culture of your environment? Think of ways in which accepted standards of practice could be enhanced. How would you bring about these vital differences?
- Identify positive attitudes towards practice in your working area. Then think about some attitudes which are not quite so positive. How would you help others to adapt their attitude in the patients' or clients' best interests?
- Identify positive leaders and leadership strategies in your practice area. How could you use these positively to play a more active leadership role in practice development?
- Do you always feel able to speak out and give your views or challenge practice decisions? If not, what situations are difficult for you, and how could you increase your assertiveness?

ONGOING PRACTICE – DISCUSSION THREE

Jasmine continued to think about ways of helping prospective patients to discuss their concerns about their imminent hospital admission. A month after the previous discussion, she met with her colleagues, Jo and Francis, to talk about their experiences.

They said they found that the new approach did not take any additional time, and they had other suggestions for how questions could be used specifically and sensitively with people who were being admitted to hospital. The main concerns for most patients seemed to be the potential length of their hospital stay and their perception of the seriousness of their planned operation.

They discussed ways of obtaining more information from the clinical areas about some of the questions patients were asking of them, and decided to ask to meet with key members of staff in these areas to gather as much useful information as possible. They also thought that perhaps they could revise the leaflets containing answers to frequently asked questions, which people could read while they were waiting for their appointment. This could help reduce the time they spent discussing common issues and allow them to focus more on patients' specific concerns and questions.

Jasmine, Jo and Francis each came away from the meeting with particular issues to follow up. They felt very confident that they could make patients' visits to the preadmission clinic as positive and as informative as possible. They felt more of a team than before because they were finding ways of working together; not just conducting appointments in their own individual ways. They also arranged follow-up meetings to continue their discussion.

How will you take the lead in making sure that change is ongoing in pursuit of excellent nursing care?

Jasmine and her colleagues were strongly motivated to enhance the patient experience at the preadmission clinic. They wanted to see each patient as an individual in their own right, which is one of the central tenets of compassionate care. They had a finite time to carry out their appointments and wanted to make best use of that time. And they wanted to prepare patients as well as they could for their admission, in order to reduce their stress and the time spent by their colleagues on the wards at the time of admission.

To enhance their service, they needed to work collaboratively, with each other and with other members of staff, on specific tasks and goals to make their vision a reality. They did not have a great deal of time at their disposal because most of their working day was spent in appointments with patients. However, some of the best advances in practice come from ideas that take very little time to implement.

The Six Seconds EQ Model (www.6seconds.org) provides a clear approach to what can be accomplished in 6 seconds. It uses the concept of emotional intelligence in relation to leadership and says that you need to:

➤ know yourself – this increases self-awareness and helps us understand what motivates others.
➤ choose yourself – act intentionally, which enables us to be problem solvers and build self-management strategies and be self-directed.
➤ give yourself – align with a common purpose, which involves putting your vision and values into action, maintaining more productive

working relationships and building thriving teams and organisations (www.6seconds.org).

It is suggested that it takes about 6 seconds for someone to recognise compassion:

> It takes six seconds to manage anger.
> It takes six seconds to create compassion.
> It takes six seconds to change the world (www.6seconds.org).

Do we always realise how important 6 seconds of our time actually is? Do we know that we can give a positive or negative impression of ourselves, or our service, in that time? We can also create a compassionate environment and make a good idea a reality in that brief period. To do so, we need to understand what constitutes a compassionate environment for our patients and clients. Identifying what is key to patients and clients feeling that they are in a compassionate environment is essential to our success. So we need to be able to define and communicate the role of compassion in nursing (Davison and Williams 2009a).

Davison and Williams (2009b) discuss the inherent difficulties of trying to measure compassion. Newton (2010) says that compassion is best taught by being a excellent role model. We have said previously that compassion might be difficult to define, 'but we know when it isn't there' (Chambers and Ryder 2009, p. 59). It is important that students, as well as being taught about the importance of compassion in the university environment, actually see it being role-modelled in their practice placements. This understanding of compassion needs to be clearly evident in student assignments, as well as their practice. Then the whole controversy of whether nurses need to be taught at degree level would be seen as irrelevant, because compassion would be perceived as integral to excellent nursing care and would be explicit. Genuine compassion mediates against compassion fatigue because the presence of compassion in nursing is motivating and stress reducing.

However, for compassion to be seen as central to excellent nursing care, there needs to be leadership and joined-up thinking. Sometimes, colleagues at ward level all have the same understanding of what constitutes excellent care – and it is shared by strategic level managers and leaders, whether they are in management, clinical specialist or education roles – but there may be no joined up thinking to ensure that the same message is conveyed vertically through educationalists to mentors to students, or through high-level managers to team leaders to nurses working with patients. In our opinion, this joined-up thinking, collaboration, leadership and theory–practice linkage needs to be a priority in all organisations.

So far in this chapter, we have discussed the potential challenges to ensuring excellence in compassionate care: resourcing, culture of the practice environment and individual nurse attitude. We have also discussed positive principles that we believe are the way to address these challenges. We now discuss actions in relation to these three challenges and suggest ways to ensure that your leadership and ability to effect change will make a real difference in patient and client experience of care. Through expert leadership, excellent and compassionate care will then become the norm in every practice area, and care that falls short of this will be challenged by all practitioners.

In terms of resourcing, these actions could include the following:

➤ Regard time and professional expertise as key resources.
➤ Make best use of time (when carrying out other tasks and interventions) to actively communicate with patients or clients.
➤ Avoid using the nursing 'minute'. Be realistic about the length of delays, or ensure that somebody else responds at the predicted time.
➤ Try to keep administrative tasks as containable as possible, and identify their impact to managers when they become too labour intensive.
➤ Use resources to as good an effect as possible.
➤ Reduce the emphasis on targets, outcomes and task-to-time ratios.
➤ Focus on what clients want and reduce what would not be missed.
➤ Remember that patients want a care provider, care partner, champion and coordinator (DOH 2008).
➤ Use bottom-up approaches to change management and the best use of resources.
➤ Minimise the impact of ineffective leadership.
➤ Maximise leadership at all levels.
➤ Focus on adopting a caring non-judgemental approach.
➤ Avoid judgemental attitudes and stereotyping.
➤ Avoid dehumanisation of patients and clients and depersonalising terminology.
➤ Communicate effectively but in shorter times; for example, brief, ordinary, effective (Wigens 2006) and solution-focused brief therapy (Berg 2003).

➤ Use emotional intelligence in improving team dynamics and keeping people feeling positive.
➤ Increase team building to improve morale, motivation and team intelligence.
➤ Reduce interpersonal conflict, because this:
 — increases staff absence and turnover
 — wastes time, money and other resources
 — leaves people feeling disempowered, disenfranchised, disengaged and marginalised.

In terms of the culture of the practice environment, the actions could include the following:
➤ Focus on maintaining a high emotional climate and temperature.
➤ Be positive, non-judgemental, appreciative and valuing to patients, clients and colleagues.
➤ Understand that we have an effect on the culture of our practice area and that this has an impact on others' beliefs and values.
➤ Realise that emotions are contagious – stay as positive as possible.
➤ Avoid being a negative role model, because negative mirroring causes a descending spiral of stress and demotivation for staff, patients and clients.
➤ Be a positive role model instead, so that positive mirroring of body language and leadership creates an ascending spiral.
➤ Help to develop a positive team culture by:
 — using personal and professional skills to best effect
 — enhancing our own motivation and nurturing that of others and being committed to high standards
 — remembering that happy and engaged staff outperform those who are not
 — ensuring that staff feel valued, respected and empowered and by giving positive feedback
 — remembering that this causes better teamwork and that people are more likely to feel in control and be change agents.
➤ Discuss what makes people feel valued and be aware of emotional touchpoints (Dewar *et al.* 2010).
➤ Encourage an environment in line with the Senses framework (Nolan *et al.* 2006) – sense of security, continuity, belonging, purpose, achievement and significance.

➤ Discuss difficult client situations.
➤ Show support of others at times of sickness, bereavement and using the '5 Whys' to get to the root of the problem (www.mindtools.com).
➤ Understand what motivates people, and work on the principle that work is natural and that people are self-directed – Theory Y (McGregor 2006).
➤ Acknowledge that some people just want to come to work and leave, while others want to develop their practice.
➤ Develop future leaders where possible.
➤ Be a visionary, transformational leader.
➤ Encourage a work–life balance.
➤ Be open and honest – develop trusting relationships and welcome challenge.
➤ Practise relational leadership based on building emotionally intelligent relationships.

In terms of personal attitudes, the actions could include the following:
➤ Avoid using inadequate resourcing as the only reason for poor standards in practice.
➤ Avoid comparisons with those who appear to practise less well.
➤ Use positive communication strategies and compassionate communication with colleagues as well as clients.
➤ Use the principles of 'See who I am, connect with me, involve me' (Nicholson *et al.* 2010a, 2010b, 2010c) with clients and colleagues.
➤ Be as personally effective as possible (Thompson 2009) – self-awareness, time management, stress management, information management, assertiveness, not accepting bullying, using supervision and CPD and being creative and realistic.
➤ Use emotional intelligence and be 'emotionally brilliant' (Goleman 1996).
➤ Use positive psychology strategies and avoid 'learned helplessness' (Seligman 1975).
➤ Find ways to reduce the effect of dissonant leaders (Goleman 2002) who focus only on pace of work and directing others.
➤ Do the same with alexithymic 'emotionally tone-deaf' personalities (Goleman 1996) who have no emotional intelligence, i.e. have feelings but do not understand them and cannot articulate them.
➤ Become a resonant leader (Goleman 2002) – there will be less emotional ill health, greater job satisfaction and collaboration.

➤ Develop personal leadership qualities of self-awareness, self-management, drive for improvement and personal integrity (NHS Leadership Qualities Framework (2006) and revised NHS Leadership Framework (2011)).

➤ Use all forms of intelligence (Furnham 2008):
   — intelligence (IQ), technical/operational (TQ), motivational (MQ), experience (XQ), people (PQ), learning (LQ) plus cultural (CQ) intelligence.

THOUGHTS FOR YOUR PRACTICE

- What is your vision for your service? How can you work collaboratively to make this vision a reality?

- Think of ways in which you demonstrate compassion in six seconds. How do you recognise this in others? Think of ways to encourage this in students and other colleagues.

- How do you know what a compassionate environment feels like for patients and clients? How do you make this a reality?

- How can you increase your focus on being an excellent role model for students and other colleagues?

- In what ways could you increase your feelings of genuine compassion to combat potential compassion fatigue? Are there any ways you could help colleagues to do the same?

- How can you ensure that students have the opportunity to experience the best care in practice? How can you design a practice curriculum that focuses on the aspects of care which patients and clients really value?

- How can you play your part in ensuring that there is joined up thinking in education and practice at all levels?

SUMMARY

Throughout the book, we have focused on the challenges, positive principles and actions that nurses can take in relation to difficult resourcing issues, attitudinal difficulties and the culture of practice environments. These can be summed up diagrammatically (*see* Figure 5.2).

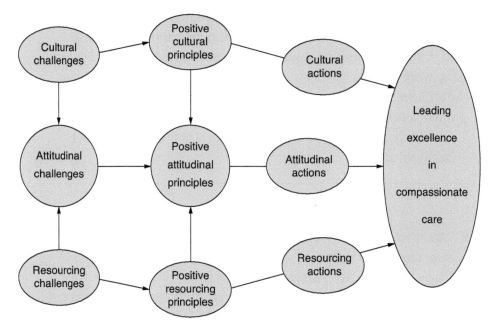

FIGURE 5.2 Key contributors to leading excellence in compassionate care

We now want to draw the discussion together by identifying the attributes of true leaders of excellent and compassionate care. In our opinion, these are (*see* Figure 5.3):

➤ personal attributes
➤ quality attributes
➤ leadership attributes
➤ educational attributes
➤ team-leading attributes.

Foster (2009) says that to energise for excellence in care, we need to ensure that the staffing is right; then we can deliver quality care, the impact of which can be measured. The result will be an enhanced patient or client experience, which in turn will mean a far better nursing experience. However, it is essential that this positive culture is led from the top and from the interface with the patients and clients we care for. Leadership needs to take place at all levels to ensure that problems are identified and solved as quickly as possible. More than that, the focus has to be on the quality of the care experience, and how we convey the importance of this to all members of our teams. These teams are multiprofessional and multifaceted; they include people who are health-care professionals, as well as those who are not. Ward clerks, receptionists,

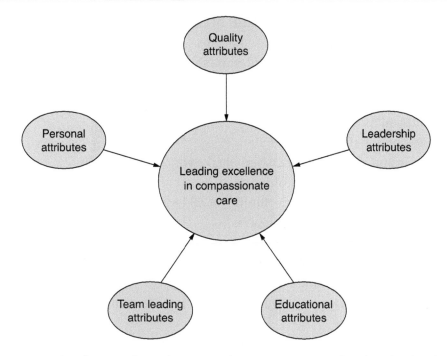

FIGURE 5.3 Leading excellence in compassionate care: personal and professional
attributes

clerks, portering staff and cleaners all contribute to the care experience, and
often acts of compassion come from those who have not had the benefit of
our education and training.

So how can we focus on our important role as leaders of excellence in compassionate care? First, by concentrating on our personal attributes, such as:

➤ emotional intelligence and emotional brilliance
➤ positive approach to practice
➤ high levels of motivation
➤ assertiveness
➤ understanding what compassion means to patients, clients and
   colleagues and conveying this to all in our team
➤ finding new ways to demonstrate compassion to patients, clients and
   colleagues.

Second, by concentrating on our quality attributes, such as:

➤ mobilising and maximising resources
➤ focusing on enhancing person-centred care
➤ challenging inappropriate resourcing

- challenging inappropriate standards of care
- challenging inappropriate cultural norms
- challenging inappropriate attitudes in others.

Third, by concentrating on our leadership attributes, such as:
- an internal locus of control
- a sense of self-efficacy
- strategic and visionary leadership – make your vision a reality
- development and support of future leaders
- maximising leadership opportunities at all levels
- making change a personal mission.

Fourth, by concentrating on our educational attributes, such as:
- compassionate role-modelling
- ensuring students and colleagues focus on excellence in practice
- positive mentoring
- teaching others about excellence and compassion
- influencing the practice curriculum of students in your practice area
- maximising education and training opportunities.

Last, by concentrating on our team-leading attributes, such as:
- developing positive team relationships
- developing positive team dynamics
- focusing on positive team communication
- maximising team skills
- enhancing team learning
- encouraging team intelligences.

Why do we need to take such a strong lead on compassion? The King's Fund report (2011) *No More Heroes* says that the heroic model of leadership, where individuals almost singlehandedly lead the organisation towards success, has been replaced by the post-heroic model of leadership. This model involves collaborative and shared leadership working formally and informally across professional boundaries. Turnbull James (2011, cited in the King's Fund report 2011, pp. 19–20) says:

> However enticing in a pressurised environment, the fantasy that getting the right leader in place will be enough to change the system, is untenable. The

healthcare context requires people who do not identify with being a leader to engage in leadership.

Leadership must be exercised across shifts 24/7 and reach to every individual: good practice can be destroyed by one person who fails to see themselves as able to exercise leadership, as required to promote organisational change, or leaves something undone or unsaid because someone else is supposed to be in charge. The NHS needs people to think of themselves as leaders not because they are personally exceptional, senior or inspirational to others, but because they can see what needs doing and can work with others to do it.

In order for us to all take this lead, we need to understand the policy drivers and evidence base for our service, and use these to point out to our senior managers what is not happening in our service. All managers tend to be risk averse, so pointing out risks and inadequacies is an important tool for us in making change happen. We might need to do this repeatedly – use adverse-incident documentation to point out institutional accountability issues – and collaborate with others to strengthen our points. Never think that you are too busy to think strategically. Identify trends and commonalities, and write emails and keep the evidence. We need to hold ourselves, and others, to account. Appraisals, clinical supervision, preceptorship, coaching and personal reflection all help us to understand the real issues in our professional lives. Occasionally, that might involve performance management with regular reviews, but usually collaborative teamworking and peer support will help others to develop their practice and identify potential problems.

We need local leaders with a clear vision, who can make that vision a reality. We need to feel empowered to make a difference, and to decide what training and education is needed to enhance care. We also need to be effective and strategic change agents who will be strong advocates for those in our care, who often cannot speak for themselves.

We are in times of great change, and in our opinion great change and challenging times need great leadership and great leaders. As we said in our first book, 'We all have a leadership role in creating a practice culture where care that lacks compassion is not tolerated and where developmental opportunities exist to enhance compassionate care' (Chambers and Ryder 2009, p. 195).

We will be happier in our personal and professional lives if we demonstrate our natural compassion. As the Dalai Lama (born 1935) says: 'If you want others to be happy, practice compassion. If you want to be happy, practice compassion.'

REFERENCES

Abraham A. *Care and Compassion? Report of the Health Service Ombudsman on Ten Investigations into NHS Care of Older People*. London: Stationery Office; 2011.

Adams C. What leadership skills will community nurses need to improve outcomes in the new NHS? *Nurs Times*. 2010; **106**(48): 10–12.

Armstrong K. *Twelve Steps to a Compassionate Life*. London: The Bodley Head; 2011.

Bailey R. In the middle of a maelstrom, good nursing is everything. *Nurs Times*. 2011; **107**(37): 11.

Berg IK. *Solution-Focused Therapy: an interview with Insoo Kim Berg*. 2003. Available at: http://psychotherapy.net/interview/Insoo_Kim_Berg (accessed 11 December 2011).

Chambers C, Ryder E. *Compassion and Caring in Nursing*. Oxford: Radcliffe Publishing; 2009.

Davison N. Williams K. Compassion in nursing 1: defining, identifying and measuring this essential quality. *Nurs Times*. 2009b; **105**(36):16–18.

Davison N. Williams K. Compassion in nursing 2: factors that influence compassionate care in clinical practice. *Nurs Times*. 2009a; **105**(37); 18–19.

Department of Health. *Confidence in Caring: a framework for best practice*. London: Department of Health; 2008.

Dewar B, Mackay R, Smith S, *et al*. Use of emotional touchpoints as a method of tapping into the experience of receiving compassionate care in a hospital setting. *J Res Nurs*. 2010; **15**(1): 29–41.

Estin N. In: Ellman M, Santos B. *Practice Aloha: secrets to living life Hawaiian style*. Hawaii: Mutual Publishing; 2010.

Foster D. Developing an effective framework to deliver nursing quality. *Second Annual Nursing Times Nursing Quality Conference Delivering High Quality Nursing Care*. 2009 Nov 18; London.

Francis R. *Independent Inquiry into Care Provided by Mid Staffordshire NHS Foundation Trust January 2005–March 2009*. Volumes 1 and 2. London: Stationery Office; 2010.

Furnham A. *Management Intelligence*. Hampshire; Palgrave Macmillan; 2008.

Goleman D. *Emotional Intelligence: why it can matter more than IQ*. London; Bloomsbury Publishing; 1996.

Goleman D. *The New Leaders*. London: Sphere; 2002.

Goodrich J. Transactional and relational aspects of care. In: Goodrich J. Understanding the patient experience of care. *Second Annual Nursing Times Nursing Quality Conference Delivering High Quality Nursing Care*. 2009 Nov 18; London.

Hodgetts S. From the top: a guide to being an effective leader. *Nurs Times*. 2011; **107**(1): 41.

Keillor G. Patient stories. 2009. In: Davies S. Compassionate care: a letter from America. *Second International Conference on Compassionate Care*. 2011 Jun 23–4; Napier University, Edinburgh.

King's Fund. *The Future of Leadership and Management in the NHS: no more heroes*. London: King's Fund; 2011.

Leitch J. Can we make compassion reliable? *Second International Conference on Compassionate Care*. 2011 Jun 23–4; Napier University, Edinburgh.

McGregor D. *The Human Side of Enterprise*. Annotated edition. New York: McGraw-Hill; 2006.

Middleton J. Walk in your patients' shoes to ensure good care. *Nurs Times*. 2011; **107**(36): 1.

Newton V. Teach students compassion by being an excellent role model. *Nurs Times*. 2010; **106**(39): 10.

Nicholson C, Flatley M, Wilkinson C, *et al*. Everybody matters 1: how getting to know your patients helps to promote dignified care. *Nurs Times*. 2010a; **106**(20): 12–14.

Nicholson C, Flatley M, Wilkinson C, *et al*. Everybody matters 2: promoting dignity in acute care through effective communication. *Nurs Times*. 2010b; **106**(21): 12–14.

Nicholson C, Flatley M, Wilkinson C. Everybody matters 3: engaging patients and relatives in decision making to promote dignity. *Nurs Times*. 2010c; **106**(22): 10–12.

Nolan M, Brown J, Davies S, *et al*. *The Senses Framework: improving care for older people through a relationship-centred approach*. Sheffield: University of Sheffield; 2006.

Pemberton M. Now I know what it's really like being an NHS patient. *Daily Telegraph*. 2010 July 5.

Prescott J. Prescott doubted 'tittle-tattle in Iraq invasion intelligence. *The Guardian*. 2010 July 30. Available at: www.guardian.co.uk/uk/2010/jul/30/john-prescott-chilcot-inquiry-testimony (accessed 22 December 2011).

Rafferty AM. We can read Nightingale as a credo for compassion today. *Nurs Times*. 2011; **107**(25): 11.

Seligman M. *Helplessness: on depression, development and death*. San Francisco, CA: WH Freeman; 1975.

Thompson N. *People Skills*. 3rd ed. Basingstoke: Palgrave Macmillan; 2009.

Turnbull James K. Leadership in context: lessons from new leadership theory and current leadership development practice. In: King's Fund. *The Future of Leadership and Management in the NHS: no more heroes*. London: King's Fund; 2011. Available at: www.kingsfund.org.uk/publications/nhs_leadership.html (accessed 22 December 2011).

Wigens L. *Communication in Clinical Settings*. Cheltenham: Nelson Thornes; 2006.

www.6seconds.org

www.mindtools.com

www.NHSLeadershipQualities.nhs.uk (2006) and revised www.nhsleadership.org.uk/framework.asp (2011).

Index

NOTE: entries in **bold** refer to figures or tables.

*9 7 8 1 8 4 6 1 9 3 9 9 6 *

An environmentally friendly book printed and bound in England by www.printondemand-worldwide.com

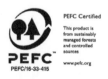

PEFC Certified

This product is
from sustainably
managed forests
and controlled
sources

www.pefc.org

PEFC/16-33-415

This book is made of chain-of-custody materials; FSC materials for the cover and PEFC materials for the text pages.

#0343 - 240216 - C0 - 246/174/10 - PB - 9781846193996